Good
TEETH

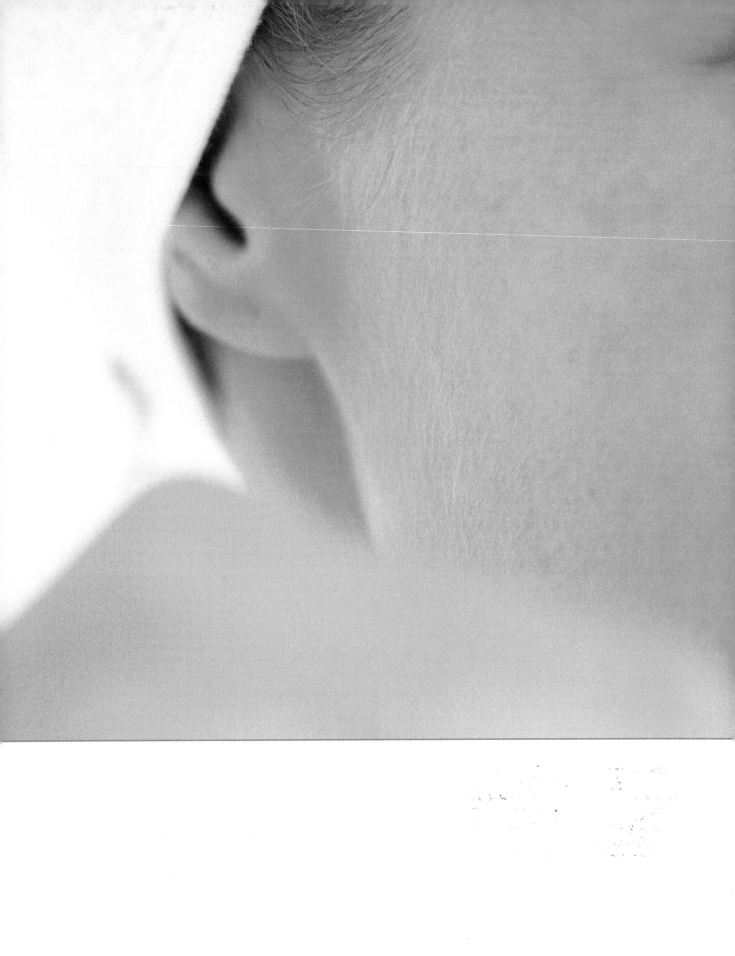

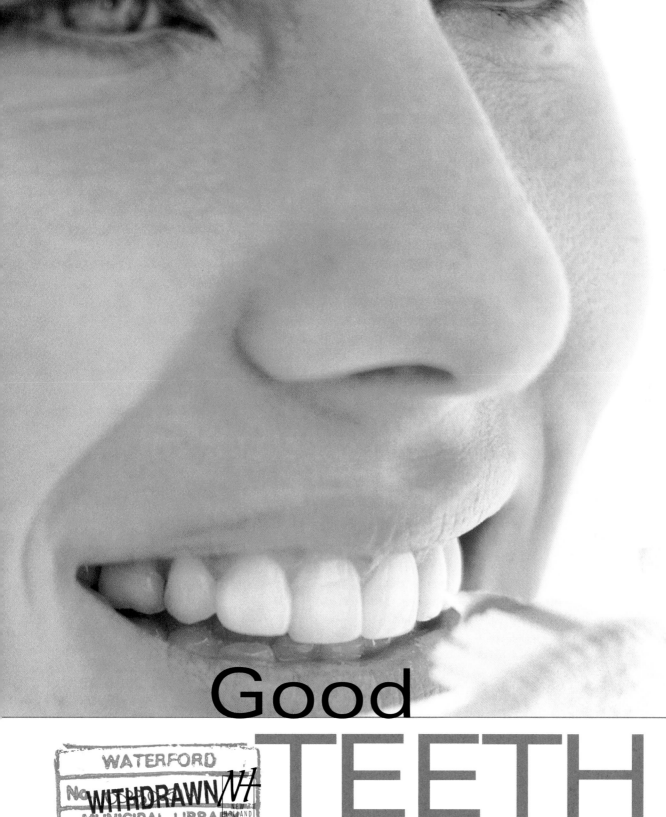

Good
TEETH

MANDY COLLINS

First published in 2005 by
New Holland Publishers
London • Cape Town • Sydney • Auckland
www.newhollandpublishers.com

86 Edgware Rd
London W2 2EA
United Kingdom

80 McKenzie Street
Cape Town 8001
South Africa

14 Aquatic Drive
Frenchs Forest
NSW 2086
Australia

218 Lake Road
Northcote
Auckland
New Zealand

Publisher: Mariëlle Renssen
Publishing managers: Claudia Dos Santos, Simon Pooley
Commissioning editor: Alfred LeMaitre
Studio manager: Richard MacArthur
Editor: Katja Splettstoesser
Concept design: Christelle Marais
Designer and illustrator: Matthew Ibbotson
Proofreader: Leizel Brown
Picture researchers: Karla Kik, Tamlyn McGeean
Production: Myrna Collins
Consultant: Dr P. Müssmann B.Ch.D(Stell), dentist in
    private practice

ISBN 1 84330 767 7 (HB); 1 84330 768 7 (PB)

Reproduction by Hirt & Carter (Cape) Pty Ltd

Printed and bound in Malaysia by Times Offset(M) Sdn. Bhd.
10 9 8 7 6 5 4 3 2 1

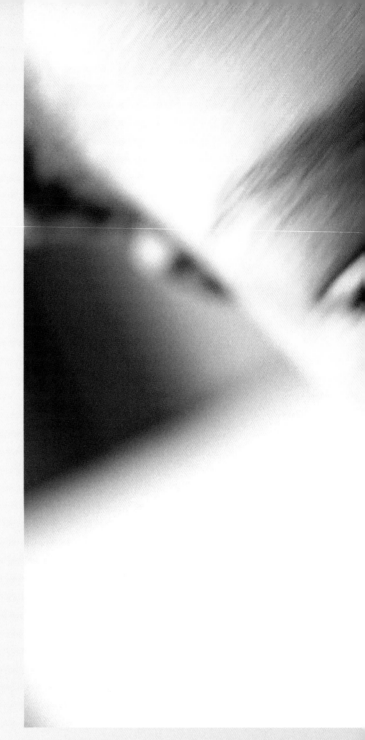

DISCLAIMER

The author and publishers have made every effort to
ensure that the information contained in this book was
accurate at the time of going to press, and accept no
responsibility for any injury or inconvenience sustained by
any person using this book or following the advice
provided herein.

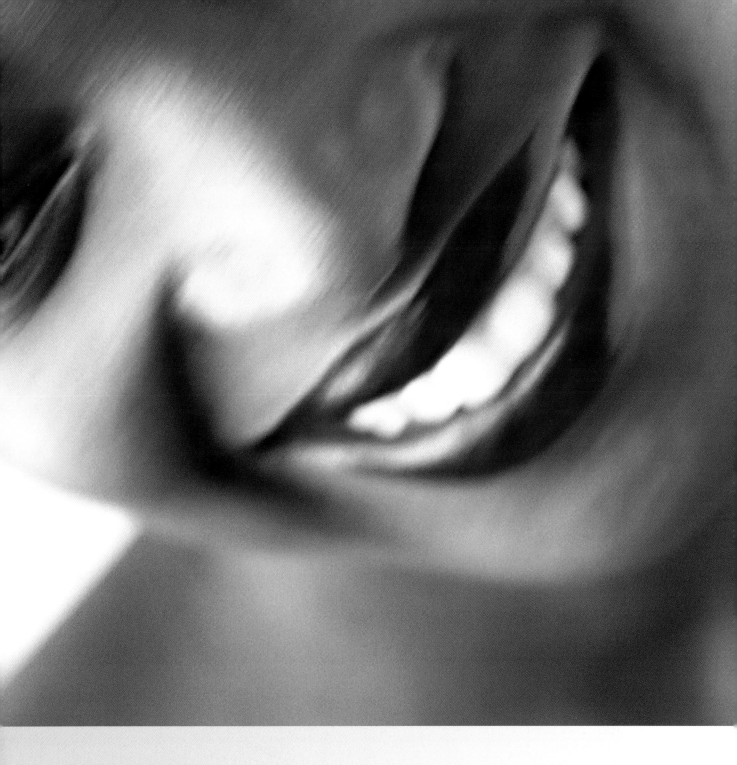

ACKNOWLEDGEMENTS

I would like to thank my husband, Rob, for his support while I wrote late into the night, as well as my daughters, Tessa and Samantha, who breathe inspiration into my life on a daily basis. I thank my parents who always encourage me in everything I tackle. Without their collective love and support, I could not have written this book. My personal 'voice of sanity', Michelle Shaw, knows just how important she is to me, as does Lynne Gidish, whose experience and professionalism have taught me a great deal. A big thank you, too, to Dr Bouke Bokma for all the information and advice, and to the South African Dental Association for filling in the gaps. Finally, Rob Sharman and Shell Paterson, thank you for instilling a love of language in me at an early age, and encouraging my early attempts at writing.

contents

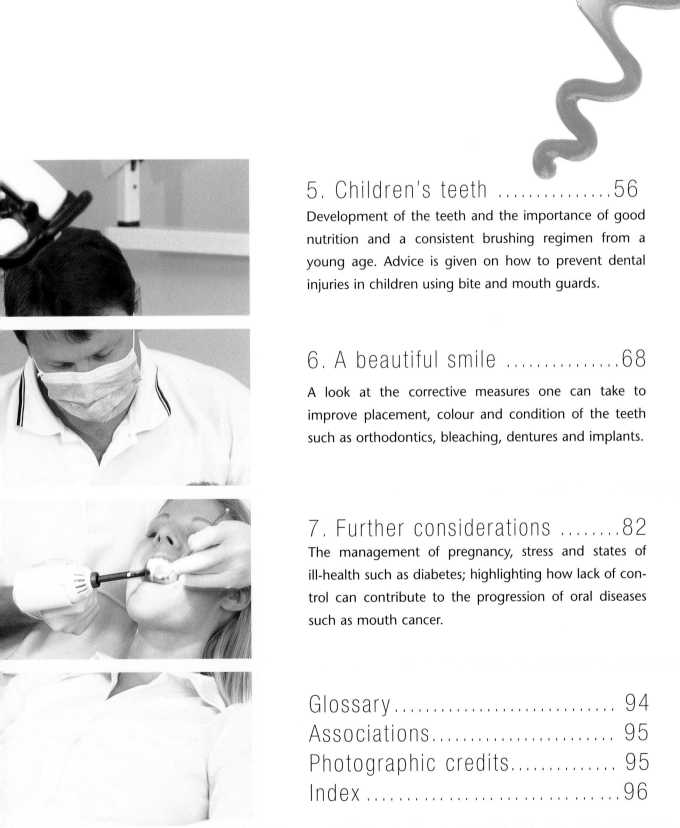

Back
to basics

We've all been brought up to brush our teeth at least twice a day and floss regularly and perhaps even use a mouthwash, but are you sure you're brushing and flossing correctly? Do you know whether or not your toothpaste is suitable for your needs? Is your toothbrush doing its job properly? The key to a healthy, beautiful smile is getting the basics right: practising the best oral hygiene you can at home, and leaving the complicated procedures to your dentist.

In addition, while most of us focus on fighting cavities, it's gum disease we should be worrying about as adults. More teeth are lost through gum disease than through tooth decay, and it is estimated that nine out of 10 people start to show signs of gum disease by the time they are 25 years old.

Fortunately, a sound oral-hygiene regimen protects your teeth against both cavities and gum disease. The key is to commit yourself to that regimen, and then implement it correctly and effectively. Doing so, just a few minutes a day, will ensure that your teeth last a lifetime.

Your teeth are supposed to last a lifetime, but cavities and gum disease are known to shorten their lifespan.

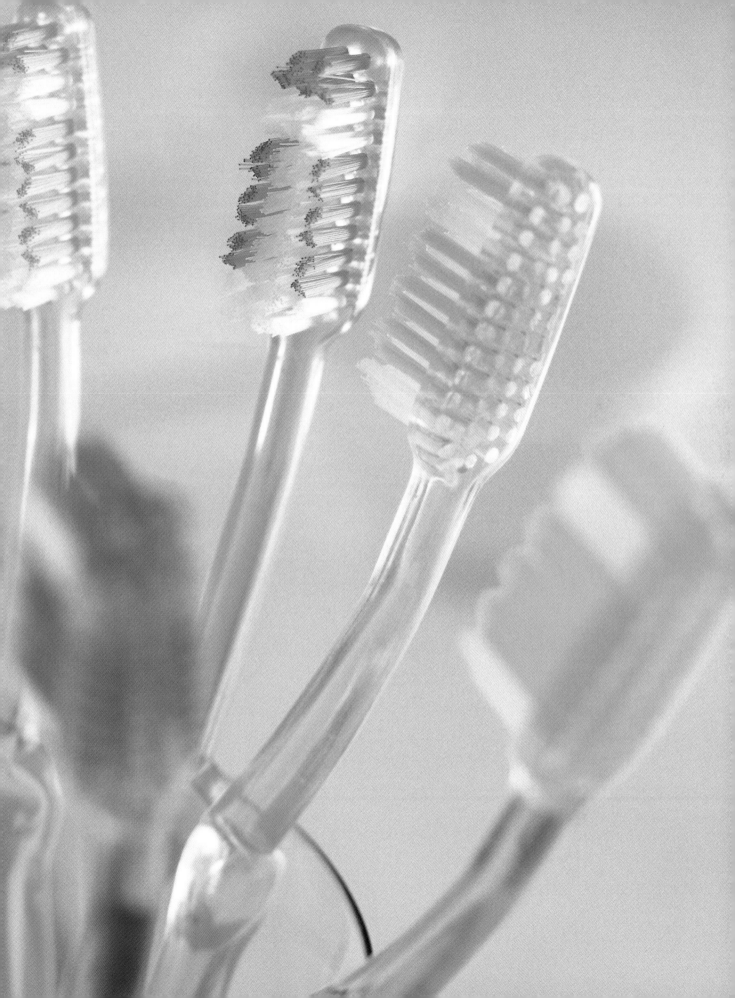

ANATOMY 101

To best understand what you're doing when taking care of your teeth, it helps to have some knowledge of their basic anatomy. Your teeth have a complex, multilayered structure, as well as a supply of nerves and blood.

The tooth is divided into three main parts: the crown, the neck and the root. Enamel covers the crown of the tooth, and this smooth, hard coating is the hardest tissue in the body. It is not sensitive at all, and is usually translucent-white in colour. The main substance of the crown, neck and root of the tooth is dentine. This is a yellow-white colour, and is very sensitive, as it houses the tooth's nerve supply.

The gums, or gingiva, are the link between the teeth and the rest of the mouth. The tiny space between the teeth and the gums is known as the gingival sulcus, and is usually no thicker than 2mm (0.08in). However, as small as it is, this space is a common source of infection. The tooth is connected to the bone in your jaw by thin fibres (periodontal ligaments), which act as shock absorbers for your teeth. The periodontal ligaments attach to the thin layer covering the root, called cementum.

ANATOMY OF A TOOTH

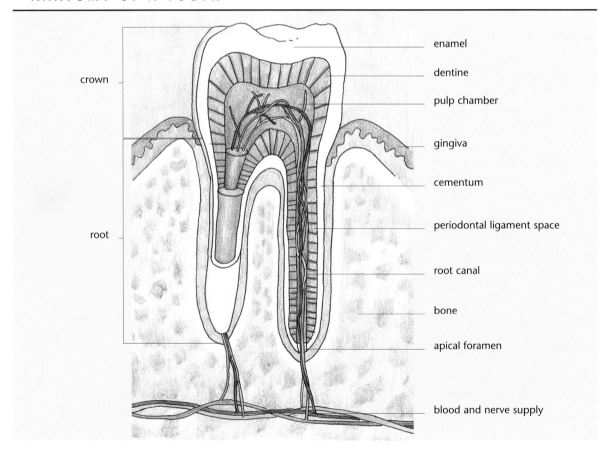

crown

root

enamel

dentine

pulp chamber

gingiva

cementum

periodontal ligament space

root canal

bone

apical foramen

blood and nerve supply

THE ORAL CAVITY

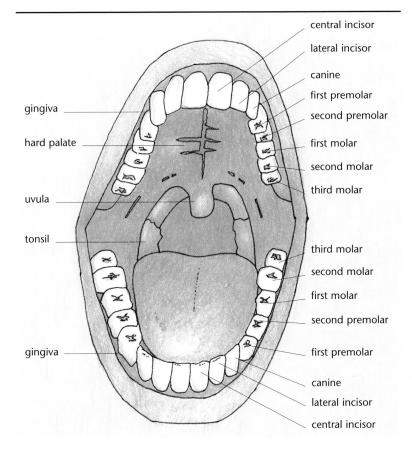

gingiva

hard palate

uvula

tonsil

gingiva

central incisor
lateral incisor
canine
first premolar
second premolar
first molar
second molar
third molar

third molar
second molar
first molar
second premolar
first premolar
canine
lateral incisor
central incisor

Inside each tooth is a nerve cavity that houses the tooth's blood vessels and nerves. Blood vessels are vital because they transport essential nutrients to the tooth, and the nerves make the tooth sensitive, which is sometimes a good thing and at other times extremely painful. The nerves and blood vessels pass through the tooth into the nerve cavity by means of small channels called root canals.

Adults have 32 teeth, including four wisdom teeth, which can be divided into four types. Each of the four types has a different structure, position and function.

The eight incisors occur near the front of the mouth, and are typically used for biting. Moving outward from the centre, your canine teeth are sharper and more pointed than incisors, and help to tear off and hold

your food while you are eating. They are also commonly called eye-teeth.

The premolars are next, and have two raised points that help to crush your food during chewing. Molars are a larger version of the premolars, and are used for grinding and pulping food. There are eight premolars and eight molars, plus the wisdom teeth that are simply an additional set of molars.

GOOD ORAL HYGIENE
Your brushing technique

Your teeth are supposed to last a life-time, but cavities and gum disease often shorten their lifespan. The key to teeth that last is correct brushing and flossing on a daily basis. Here, prevention really is better than cure.

However, while we all probably brush our teeth at least once daily, and floss occasionally, the question is whether or not we are brushing

The key to teeth that will last is correct brushing and flossing daily.

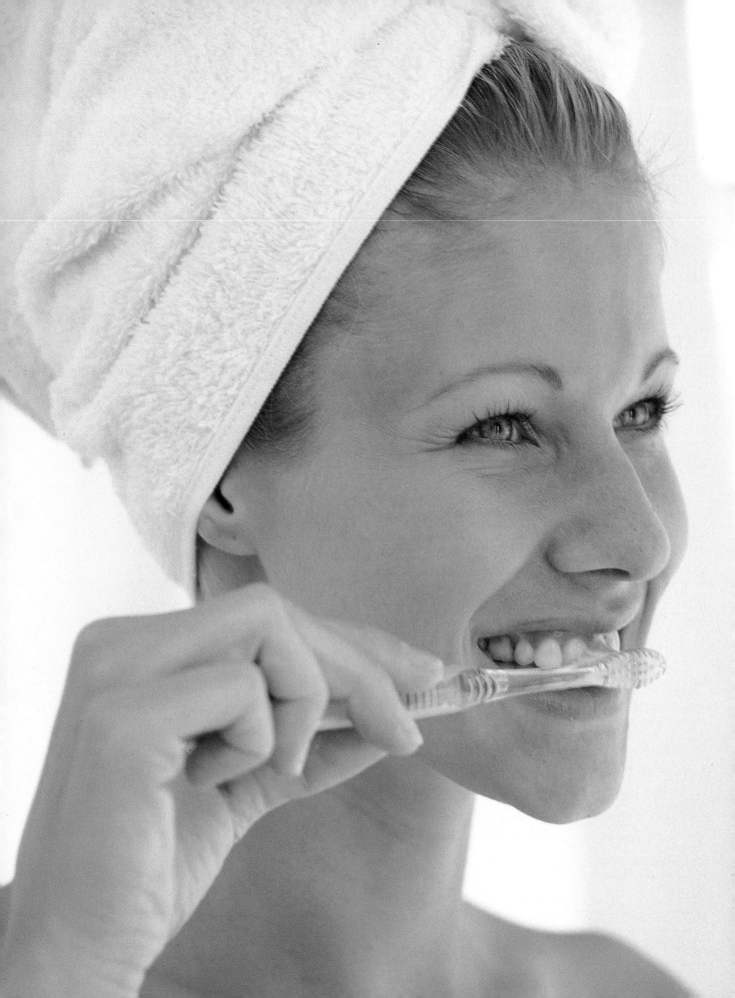

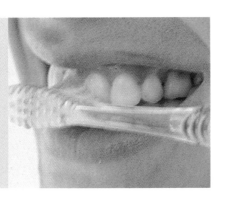

Ensure you are holding your toothbrush firmly, but comfortably, with its head at a slight angle to your teeth, and systematically clean every surface.

correctly and effectively. A good brushing technique is vital if you are going to get into all the nooks and crannies between tooth and gum. So here's a basic guideline: hold the toothbrush in a comfortable grip and place the head at about 45 degrees to the surface of your teeth: this allows the bristles to get into the space between the gum and teeth. Starting at one side of your mouth, systematically brush first the outside of your upper and lower teeth, moving from one side of your mouth to the back of the other side. Then do the same for the inside of all the teeth, working from one side to the other, and repeat for the chewing surfaces.

Finally, wipe your tongue with two or three strokes from back to front, and use your tongue to test whether or not your teeth feel smooth and clean. If not, return to whichever areas need attention, and brush them again.

In the absence of fluoridated water, it is essential to use a toothpaste containing fluoride. Note that, unlike adults, if children ingest too much fluoride, it can discolour their teeth, so you need to find a good balance.

Fluoride strengthens their teeth in two ways: either from the inside, where it is systemically absorbed, or by direct application to the surfaces of teeth to make them more resistant to decay. The latter is what you are doing when you brush your teeth.

To get the balance right, start by brushing your teeth at least twice a day – three times if you can manage it. If you really can't get that right, then at least ensure that your once-a-day brushing occurs last thing at night. Bacteria accumulate on your teeth during the day, and saliva flow diminishes at night, so your teeth have less protection while you sleep. When you have finished brushing your teeth, don't rinse your mouth afterwards – simply spit out any excess toothpaste and leave the remainder on your teeth, so that the fluoride can do its work.

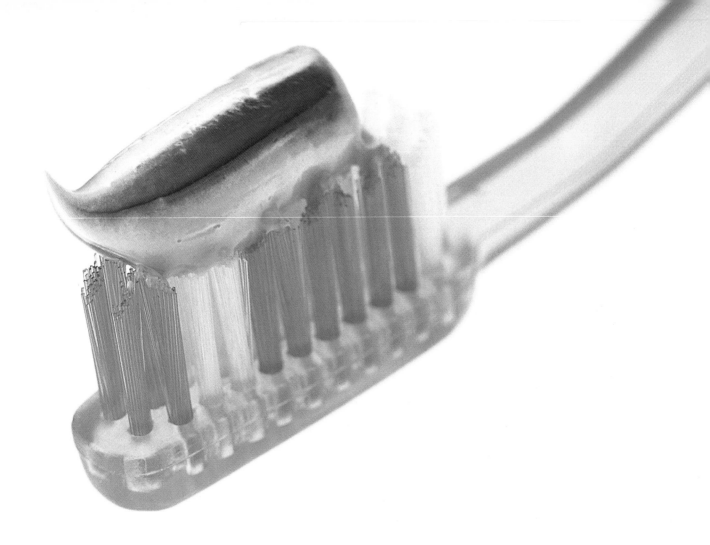

Choosing a toothbrush

Part of effective brushing is having a good toothbrush. Many people think that to do the job properly they need a good, hard brush, but in fact, all they are doing with a hard brush is damaging the enamel of their teeth and bruising their gums.

There are basic requirements for a good toothbrush: its head should not be longer than 20mm (0.8in). It

should also have nylon bristles that are medium-soft rather than hard, and its tips should be rounded. While it may seem unimportant, a comfortable grip makes a huge difference. If your hand slips while brushing, you can injure your gums or palate, so it's worth finding a brush that is both comfortable to hold and unlikely to become slippery when wet.

Another option is the power or electric toothbrush: most dentists tell you that advances in this area have revolutionized how well we are able to brush our teeth at home. Power toothbrushes clean your teeth much better than you ever could, and are very gentle on the gums. Some people might find the sensation a little strange at first, as they vibrate fast, but once you've been using a power toothbrush for a while, a manual toothbrush simply won't seem to do the job well enough.

Power toothbrushes have been scientifically proven to modestly reduce plaque, gingivitis and secondary gum disease, which make them a good bet. They leave your teeth feeling fresher, smoother and cleaner than a manual toothbrush would. Remember, however, that they do not take away the need to have your teeth professionally cleaned by an oral hygienist as tartar cannot be effectively removed with either a manual or power toothbrush.

If you decide a power toothbrush is for you, here's a valuable tip: don't switch it on until it's in your mouth, or you will be mopping up toothpaste splatters on every surface in your bathroom! Also avoid using tooth-whitening toothpaste with an electric toothbrush; the combination is too abrasive and you may damage your teeth's surface enamel.

Electric toothbrushes are expensive and this is a major drawback for most people. The initial outlay is steep, but then it's not necessary to buy one for every member of the family. Most people buy one brush for the family, plus a multipack of refill heads: these usually come in packs of four, and each head has its own marker and colour. Each family member then simply puts on his or her own toothbrush head when they want to brush their teeth.

There are excellent electric toothbrushes on the market; find out from your dentist which brand is best, if this is something you would like to try. Whatever toothbrush you choose

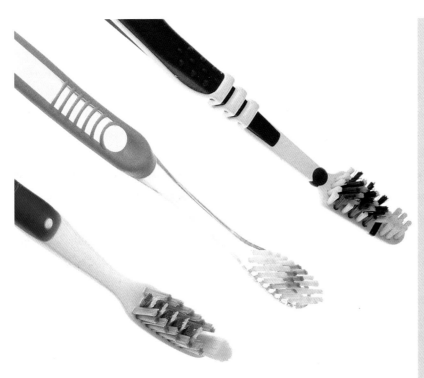

SELECTING TOOTHBRUSHES

WHAT TO LOOK FOR:
- The head should be no more than 20mm (0.8in) long.
- The nylon bristles should be medium-soft.
- The bristles should have rounded tips.
- The grip should be comfortable and nonslip.

15

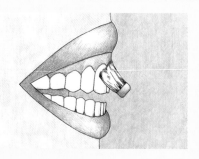

Hold a toothbrush at 45 degrees to the chewing surfaces of your teeth; brush in a gentle circular movement.

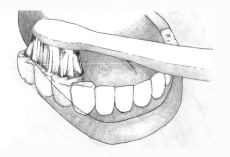

Brush the chewing surfaces of your molars with extra care.

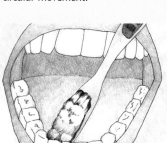

Don't forget to brush behind your teeth to remove plaque.

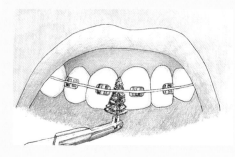

If you wear braces, an interdental brush will allow you to get in behind them.

to use, remember that it won't last forever. Some toothbrushes have coloured bristles that fade to white when it's time to get a new one; otherwise, a good guideline is to buy a new brush every six weeks, or more often if it's starting to look worn. Note that your toothbrush is a weapon for fighting plaque build-up and oral disease, so it's vital that you get the best possible brush on the market.

Mouthwashes

While brushing and flossing are the cornerstones of good oral hygiene, a mouthwash is a useful addition to your tooth-cleaning regimen. Rinsing your mouth out thoroughly can help to prevent bacteria from accumulating there, causing gum disease and other oral infections.

Often, an antibacterial mouthwash gets into places your toothbrush and dental floss can't reach. Some can even loosen plaque, while most at least give you a fresh-smelling breath. Mouthwashes vary in flavour and effectiveness, and some even treat mild throat infections, although these are best used only when you need them. If you want to use a mouthwash, find one that offers antibacterial properties and has a flavour you are able to face day after day.

Flossing

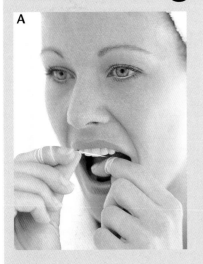
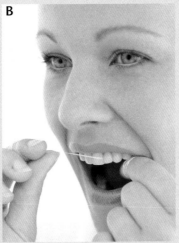
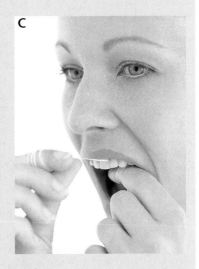

Flossing is one of those areas where many of us need improvement. It can seem like too much of an effort to floss when all you want to do is brush your teeth and fall into bed at the end of a long day.

Flossing, however, is one of the most common and effective ways of getting rid of plaque and food debris between your teeth; that's why your dentist or oral hygienist flosses your teeth at every visit.

There are many kinds of dental floss on the market, so if you are at a loss as to which one to use, consult your dentist, or try a few different brands until you find one that works well for your teeth. Also ensure you are using the correct technique, as flossing incorrectly can actually damage your teeth. Again, your dentist or oral hygienist can help you here, and demonstrate correct techniques if necessary. Here's a basic guide:

Cut off a good length of dental floss, about 50cm (20in), and twist it around the middle or index fingers of both your hands, so that you have about 10cm (4in) of floss pulled tightly between your hands (A). Supporting the floss with your index fingers or thumbs, guide it between the teeth, and use a gentle sawing motion to move it back and forth from the base of the tooth to its crown (B). Take care when pulling the floss: use your other teeth to support your fingers as you can cut your gums if your hand slips.

It's vital that when you insert the floss between your teeth you curve it into an arc around one tooth, which you clean thoroughly, and then clean the adjoining surface of the adjacent tooth (C). Don't simply place the floss between your teeth and slide it to and fro. You need to ensure you clean each tooth individually.

Common
oral problems

There is more to preserving your teeth than correct brushing and flossing. Sometimes, in spite of our best efforts, we still get cavities or suffer from gum disease. In fact, the latter is more of a problem than most of us realize: gum disease is by far the biggest cause of tooth loss in adults.

Cleaning your teeth properly plays a huge part in preventing problems such as cavities or gum disease, but it's not always enough. Other factors like diet, lifestyle and even your genetic make-up all play a role in the state of your teeth and gums. Also, broadly speaking, children and adults fall into different risk groups.

Diet, lifestyle and your genetic make-up all play a role in the state of your teeth and gums.

Because you can't guarantee perfect oral health through your own efforts alone, you need to visit your dentist twice a year. While most people only ever suffer from cavities, you need to be aware that there are more serious oral conditions such as cancer, that might require early treatment if they are to be controlled. For this reason, it's important to report any changes in your mouth to your dentist as soon as you notice them.

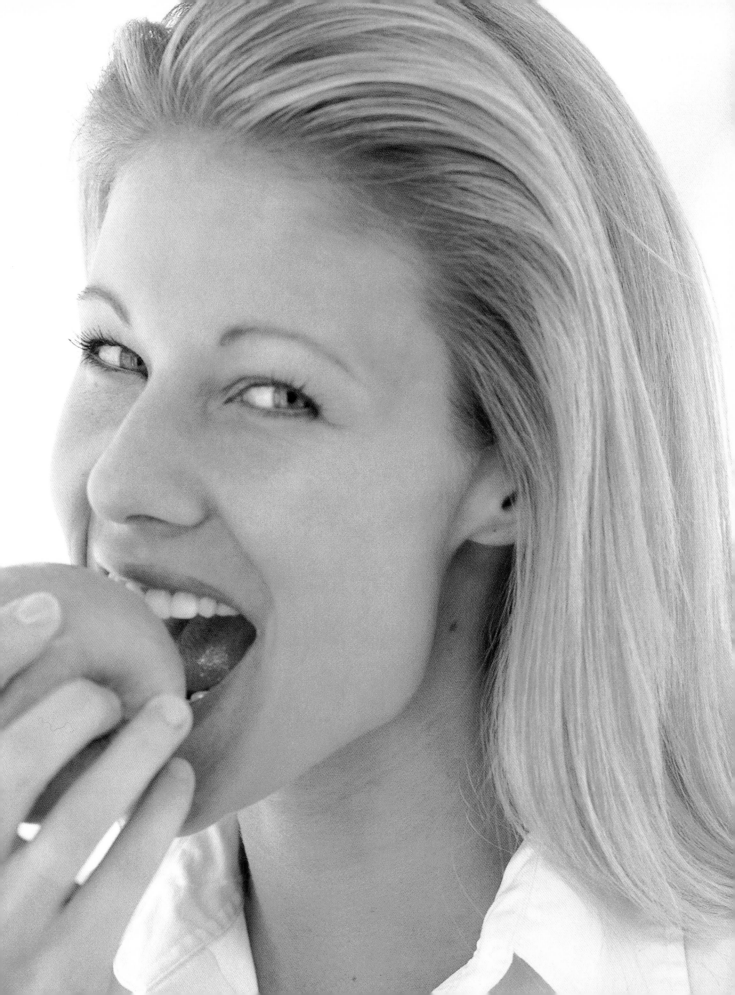

Tooth decay

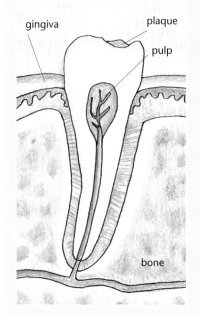

gingiva
plaque
pulp
bone

Without thorough regular flossing and brushing, plaque deposits begin to accumulate on and around the tooth. Acids form and start to decalcify the enamel, making it softer and more susceptible to decay.

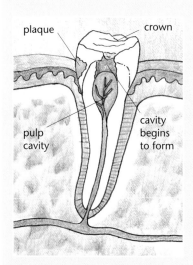

plaque
crown
pulp cavity
cavity begins to form

The tooth decalcifies right down to the dentine and becomes sensitive to cold and sweet food.

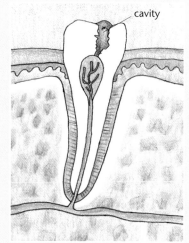

cavity

The caries goes into the nerve; the tooth becomes sensitive to hot food and may become infected.

TOOTH DECAY

Tooth decay, or dental caries, has been around for centuries: ancient Neanderthal skulls confirm this. It's also the most common disease in the world today. Decay poses the biggest threat to children's teeth, but that doesn't mean adults are exempt from this disease; their risk is just lower after age 20.

To understand tooth decay, you need to understand plaque: a combination of saliva, normal oral bacteria and food particles in the mouth that sticks to the teeth. All three factors (saliva, bacteria and food particles) have to be present for plaque to form, and it takes a few hours to accumulate. Once plaque starts to form, the bacteria in it produce organic acids that eat away at the hard tissue of the tooth, and you have the beginnings of a cavity.

Once the acids start to decalcify the surface of the tooth, the enamel in the area becomes softer and chalk-white in colour. This is the first sign of caries. The bacteria and acids are then able to move into the decalcified part of the tooth, and continue damaging it at a deeper level. At this stage, plaque has entered the tooth, and can no longer be removed by brushing.

A dentist can still, however, remove the affected part and stop the process by inserting a filling.

Should the disease progress further with no intervention from a dentist the tooth will decalcify until the decay reaches the dentine, at which stage it becomes sensitive to cold and sweet stimuli such as food.

The next stage is when the decay penetrates deeper into the dentine and approaches the nerve. Your tooth then becomes sensitive to hot food and drinks. Next, it spreads into the nerve chamber, which can cause infection. This is because of the direct opening that leads from the mouth, through and into the inner part of the tooth that is normally protected. It's a bit like an open wound on the skin, except, in this case, it is the inner cavity of your tooth that's exposed and infected. This infection may lead to the formation of an abscess (a localized collection of pus) in the tooth, or even in the bone, or tissue, around the tooth. By this stage you are in agony, and saving the tooth involves removal of the nerve, commonly known as a root-canal treatment. This whole process, from decalcification of the enamel to penetration of the nerve chamber, takes no less than 12 months.

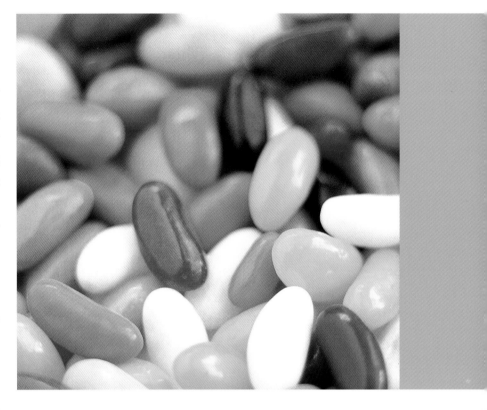

Clearly, from the above explanation, food particles are the catalyst in this process. If they are removed, by means of brushing or flossing, plaque formation can easily be prevented. Also, while conventional wisdom says that sugar is the main culprit in causing tooth decay, it is in fact all carbohydrates that contribute to the formation of plaque and cavities because they convert to acid more readily than other foods do.

The secret behind minimizing the effects of carbohydrate-rich food is to

Brightly coloured sweets such as these jellybeans look irresistible, but their high sugar content can cause great damage to your tooth enamel.

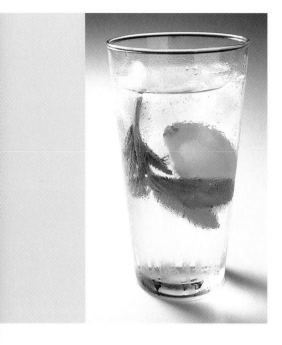

ABOVE: *A glass of water is always a healthier choice of drink than a sugary drink or even fruit juice.*
OPPOSITE: *There is nothing better than an ice-cream on a hot day, but try to brush your teeth afterwards, if possible.*

As a guideline, the stickier the food, the worse it is for your teeth.

cut down the number of times you eat carbohydrates a day. Eating carbohydrates less often means there is less acid in contact with your teeth, and therefore, fewer occurrences of cavities. Some dentists suggest cutting sugar out of your diet and replacing it with artificial sweetener. This is, however, an idealistic expectation because when people cut sugar out of their diet, they tend to increase their fat intake; not a good option for their general health and wellbeing.

A more realistic way of dealing with carbohydrates is to ensure you eat them less frequently – a maximum of five times a day would suffice – and to be aware of what you snack on between meals. Also, if possible, try to brush your teeth after eating carbohydrates.

As a guideline, the stickier the food, the worse it is for your teeth.

There's also some bad news, however: despite your best efforts to follow these guidelines, you may simply be more susceptible to caries than others. Some people seem to be able to eat what they like – while those who are more at risk, probably as a result of their genetic make-up, may find that even reducing their

carbohydrate intake doesn't help. It's here that one has to go a step further, and make use of fluoride to help strengthen your teeth.

The role of fluoride has varied over the years. Taken internally, it does significantly reduce the incidence of caries, and its introduction into toothpaste has made a difference to the number of tooth-decay cases dentists are seeing. However, if you are planning to take fluoride supplements, ensure you do so under the guidance of your dentist, as too much fluoride can leave white-and-brown flecks and even slight depressions on your teeth.

The issue of fluoridating water is a controversial one. Many countries around the world have introduced fluoridated water, but many people object to this practice on the grounds that they are being 'medicated' against their will. However, despite some debate as to what concentration of fluoride gives the best results, there's no doubt that the fluoride content of water has a significant bearing on the non-prevalence of caries.

It's not really in the scope of this book to get into the fluoride debate, but if you are contemplating taking fluoride supplements, you should definitely not do so if the water in your

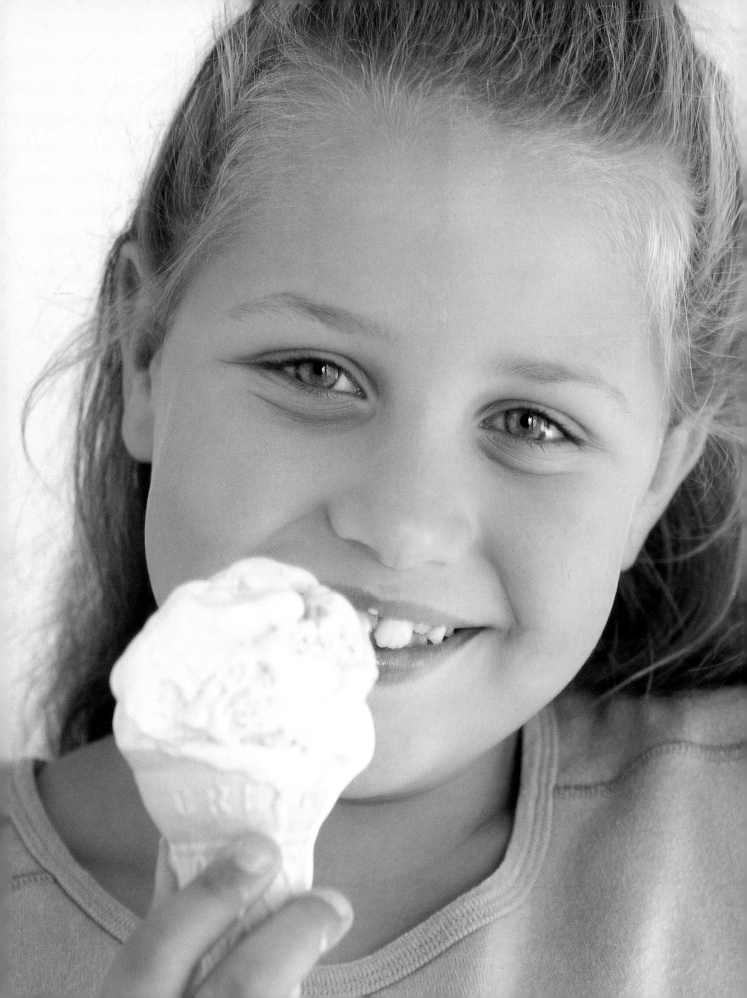

area is fluoridated. As an aside: there are other benefits to fluoridating drinking water: following the introduction of fluoridated water in Grand Rapids, Michigan in 1995, it was found to reduce the level of osteoporosis among those who drank it!

Note: If the water in your area *is* fluoridated, and you don't want to ingest fluoride this way, drink bottled mineral water, or invest in a water purifying system for your home: either have a device fitted to your kitchen tap or purchase a water-filtering jug.

GUM DISEASE

After the age of 35, gum disease or periodontitis is the major cause of tooth loss in adults, far more so than tooth decay. In fact, about 80 per cent of tooth loss can be ascribed to periodontal disease in this age group. A lot of time and money could be saved by early detection and treatment of the disease and many more people would keep their teeth if they were aware of this fact.

Periodontal disease affects the supporting structures of the teeth: the bone, gums and ligaments. It is a long-term and slow-moving disease: painless in its initial stages, but later presenting as a chronic inflammation that damages both the gums and bone holding the teeth in place. Bacterial plaque is the main culprit here, and only fastidious daily brushing and flossing can effectively remove it.

When plaque is not properly removed from the teeth, the millions of bacterial organisms in it combine with some constituents of saliva to

THE PROGRESSION OF PERIODONTITIS

EARLY PERIODONTITIS

Tartar on the tooth, which is a deposit of calcified plaque containing toxins and bacteria, infects the adjoining gums and causes them to become more inflamed with time. Here, the gum has receded 2mm (0.08in), as shown by the periodontal probe, used by dentists to test for periodontitis, and there is the onset of damage to the tooth's bone and ligament.

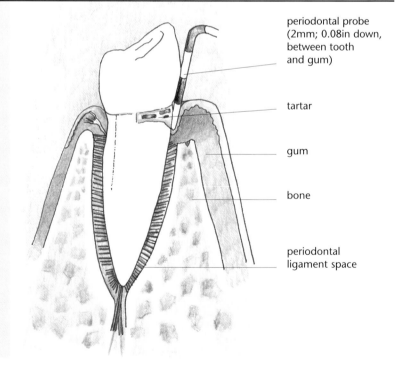

periodontal probe (2mm; 0.08in down, between tooth and gum)

tartar

gum

bone

periodontal ligament space

INTERMEDIATE PERIODONTITIS

The gums become even more inflamed, and with the periodontal ligament now seriously damaged by the infection, bone loss starts in earnest.

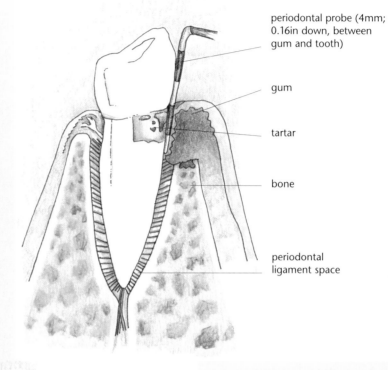

periodontal probe (4mm; 0.16in down, between gum and tooth)

gum

tartar

bone

periodontal ligament space

periodontal probe (6mm (0.24in) down, between gum and tooth)

gum

bone

periodontal ligament space

ADVANCED PERIODONTITIS

The teeth become loose because the supporting tissue around them has been too badly damaged. This is the most advanced stage. At this stage the teeth can no longer be saved, and will have to be removed.

	SYMPTOMS	LOCAL FACTORS	TREATMENT
GINGIVITIS	• Swollen gums that bleed frequently and easily • Shiny, bright red or red-purple gums • Little, or no discomfort • May have sores (ulcers)	• Micro-organisms • Tartar • Food impaction • Faulty restorations • Chemicals and drugs	• Can be reversed • Proper brushing and flossing essential • Treatment by a dentist or oral hygienist to remove tartar and control plaque.
PERIODONTITIS	• Bleeding gums during and after brushing • Red, swollen, tender gums • Bad breath • Bad taste in mouth • Receding gums • Loose or shifting teeth • Visible pockets between teeth and gums	**SYSTEMIC FACTORS** • Nutritional imbalance • Drug action • Pregnancy, diabetes and endocrine dysfunctions • Allergies • Hereditary factors • Immunopathies	• Healthy eating • Correct brushing and flossing; power toothbrushes • Anti-bacterial toothbrushes and mouthwashes • Scaling and root planing • Surgery • Antibiotics • Bone and soft-tissue grafts

Gingivitis develops into periodontitis that involves the gums, alveolar bone, cementum and periodontal ligament.

form a hard porous deposit called tartar. Not only does the tartar cause more irritation and infection, but toxins from the bacteria destroy the supporting tissues of the teeth.

As a result, the gums pull away from the teeth, forming pockets which fill with more plaque. The pockets grow deeper as the disease progresses: plaque moves further down the roots, and more bone loss occurs. The damage may be permanent if not treated in time.

The warning signs of gum disease begin with swollen, red gums that bleed easily. Ironically, many people believe that it's normal for their gums to bleed, which is most definitely not the case, as bleeding is usually a sign of underlying disease.

In the beginning stages you won't feel any discomfort or pain, which is why so many people leave treating it until it's too late. Left untreated, periodontitis causes irreversible damage, so it's vital to pay attention to the health of your gums on a daily basis, and to visit your dentist if you notice any changes.

While plaque is the main cause of gum disease, there are other factors to consider, all of which affect the health of your gums: diet, smoking, stress, diseases like leukaemia and HIV/AIDS in their latter stages, pregnancy, and medication such as oral contraceptives. Even anti-depressants and some heart and anti-convulsive medication may all have an adverse effect on gum health. Don't forget your genetic make-up: your parents' oral health may well give you clues as to what to expect from your teeth and gums as you grow older.

Your dentist makes a point of checking the state of your gums when you go for your biannual visits.

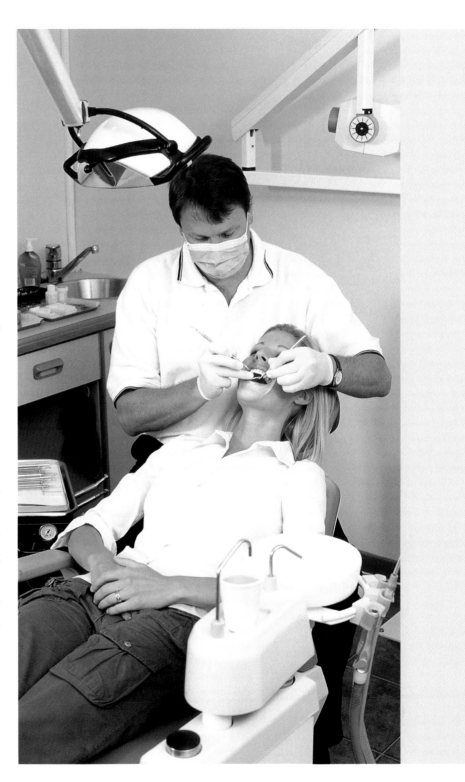

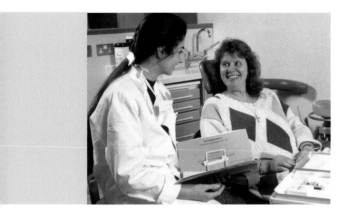

Visiting your dentist is not just about looking for cavities. Controlling gum disease is a vital part of the dental consultation, because it is a common problem in adults.

While periodontal disease is treatable, again prevention is a key factor. So it's back to the basics of brushing and flossing correctly, as that keeps the formation of tartar to a minimum. However, be aware that no matter how con-scientious you are, you're unlikely to get rid of all of the plaque and tartar as there are some places your tooth-brush and dental floss just can't reach! This makes those twice-yearly visits to the dentist and oral hygienist of paramount importance because they have the tools and expertise to make sure that all the surfaces on your teeth are clean.

Diagnosis and treatment

Gum disease is diagnosed by testing the colour and firmness of your gums, checking for gum pockets and assessing the mobility of your teeth. A change in the way you bite over a period of time may also be a symp-tom of periodontal disease.

Treatment starts with scaling and root planing: your dentist or hygienist uses an ultrasonic machine that 'vibrates' the tartar off the teeth.

Hand-held instruments are then used to smooth the roots. These two steps remove most of the bacteria, and allow the gums to adapt themselves back to the teeth, or at least to shrink enough to eliminate the pockets that have formed.

If you have more advanced gum disease, however, surgical inter-vention may be a means to radically slow its progress and hopefully pre-vent any further activity. Depending on the severity of your symptoms, you may be sent to a specialist who treats gum disease on a regular basis.

Surgery is performed either under general anaesthetic, or in the den-tist's chair under local anaesthetic: your dentist will discuss which options are best for your particular case. The aim of the surgery is to remove tartar from the deep pockets in the gums, and to reduce their appearance by means of plastic surgery. The surgical techniques involved rearrange the gum tissue into a shape that is easy to clean. Damaged bone can also be surgically re-contoured, and in very advanced cases, the teeth are propped up with temporary splints.

There are also some other possible treatments, all dependent on the stage of the disease and the damage that has occurred. These include bite adjustment, orthodontic treatment, the use of a retainer and even antibiotics, although these procedures must be combined as they are not effective in isolation.

Unfortunately, gum disease, more often than not, is controlled rather than cured, just as one controls diabetes or high blood pressure. So it's vital, if you are diagnosed and treated for gum disease, that you enrol yourself in a maintenance programme that allows your dentist or specialist to monitor your dental health closely. This also means visiting an oral hygienist regularly every six weeks to three months and ensuring your brushing and flossing techniques are correct.

If you don't control your gum disease at an early stage, you stand to lose all your teeth: not a path most of us want to follow. The benefits of retaining your natural teeth cannot be underestimated: comfortable chewing, better digestion and a healthy smile, the latter being an important asset to your appearance. Most importantly, you avoid the pain and discomfort associated with periodontal disease.

ABSCESSES

There are many causes of dental abscesses and you won't always know you have one, because while acute abscesses develop quite quickly and are painful, chronic abscesses may not be painful at all.

Acute abscesses are painful because the abscess causes swelling, and there is no room inside or around the tooth to accommodate that swelling. When there is infection in the body, it is normal to experience a degree of swelling as a result of fluid build-up in the area. When that fluid is unable to escape, the result is pain.

The reason chronic abscesses may not be sore is that this fluid has managed to develop an escape route. This allows it to drain, relieving pressure in the area, thus you don't feel any pain, or, if you are experiencing pain, it is likely to be minor.

Your dentist treats an abscess in a number of different ways, depending on where it is located, and what it has affected. The key, however, is to remove the source of the infection and drain the abscess. This may involve root-canal treatment, periodontal reparation, or even removal of the tooth and the prescription of an antibiotic to remove any infection.

If you don't do anything to control gum disease, you stand to lose your teeth.

The dentist

The dentist is your ally in keeping your mouth and teeth healthy, so it's vital you find someone you trust, and can consult routinely every six months. You may need to see him more often if you have a dental problem that needs follow-up treatment or long-term care, but generally, most people see their dentists twice a year for a checkup, or the odd filling or root-canal treatment.

The reason it's important to see your dentist regularly every six months is to identify and diagnose problems at an early stage. Teeth do not heal in the way that injured skin does, for example, so if you have a problem, only your dentist can identify it and treat it, as it will not clear up by itself. Any damage to your teeth or gums is irreversible, so it's vital you get expert help.

Any damage to your teeth or gums is likely to be irreversible, so it's vital you get expert help.

Unless you've been going to the same person for many years, finding a dentist is not easy, particularly if you move to a new town or your dentist has retired. In these cases you will need to find someone who delivers both quality oral healthcare, and with whom you have a good rapport.

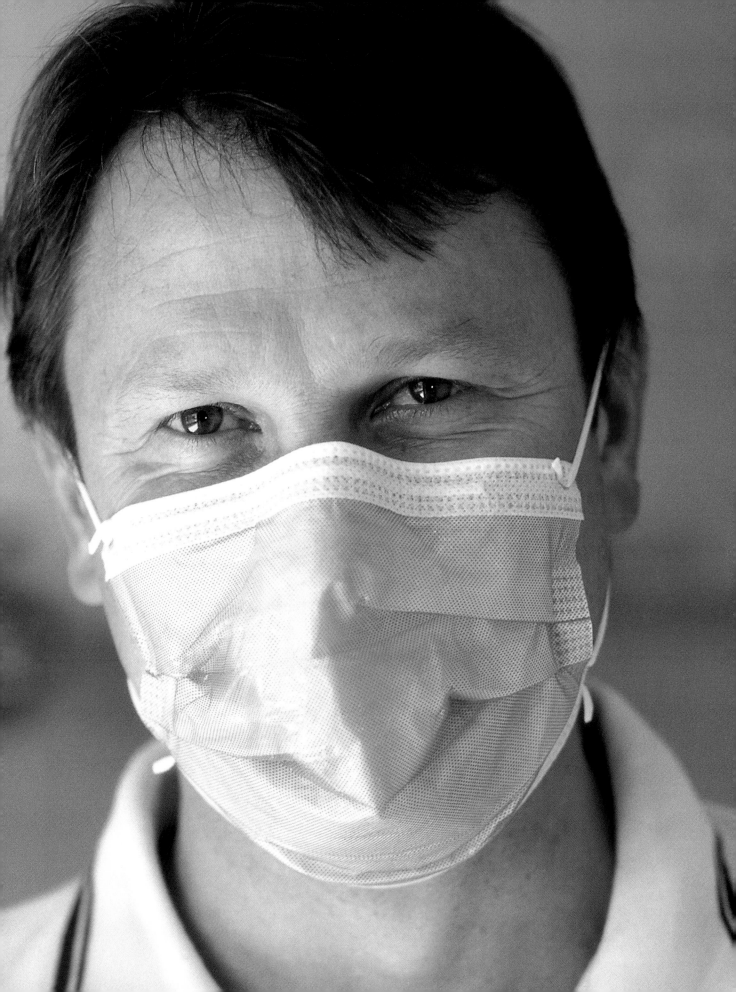

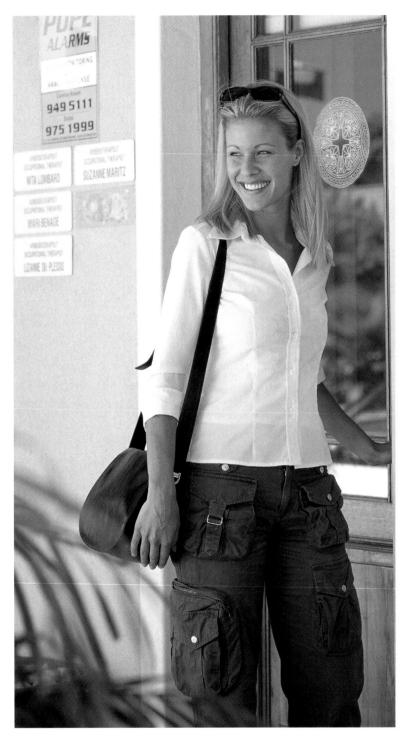

Regular visits to the dentist will ensure that you can smile with confidence.

CHOOSING A DENTIST

If you consult your dentist regularly, then it's probably someone you've been seeing for a long time and trust completely to take good care of your oral health. If you have been avoiding the dentist for many years, however, or have recently moved to a new town, you may find yourself in a position where you know you need to find a suitable dentist, but do not have a clue as to how to choose this particular person.

Rather than picking someone at random, it's best in this situation to speak to friends and to get a referral from someone you trust, preferably someone who feels the same way you do about going to the dentist. Your doctor, or even a dental specialist, may also be a good place to find out about a reputable dentist in your area. Dental specialists such as orthodontists and maxillo-facial surgeons deal with dentists on a daily basis, and know who's doing a good job, and who is not.

Before you book your appointment and seat yourself in the dentist's chair, ensure you have chatted to the person concerned, and communicated any expectations and fears you might have. You should feel completely comfortable asking whatever questions you

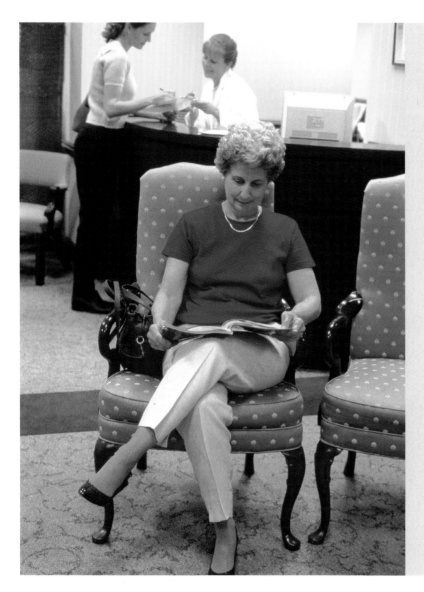

Use the time spent in the dentist's waiting room to take your mind of the impending procedure, and do something relaxing if you feel anxious about your visit.

may have about your treatment. Having this chat is important, as you will be able to determine whether or not you are likely to have a rapport with the dentist you've chosen, and are comfortable with his or her philosophy of treatment.

Also discuss costs: you need to ensure, firstly, that your new dentist understands what your budgetary constraints are, and secondly, that the services offered match the price being charged. Most countries have a dental association or society of some sort that

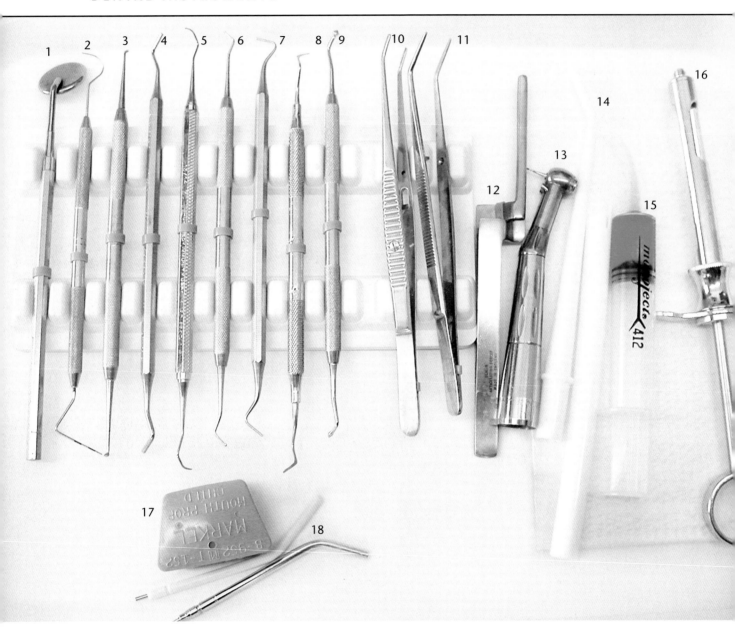

Dental practitioners ensure they always use high quality, well maintained instruments such as these (from left to right): Mirror (1), Pr (2), Carver (3), Chisel (4), Gracey curette (5), Excavator (6), Plugger (7), Carver (8), Burnisher (9), Locking college tweezer (10), Co tweezer (11), Biting paper holder (12), Air turbine (drill) (13), Suction tips (14), Syringe (15), Breech-locking syringe (16), Rubber bi block (17) and 3-in-1 syringe tips (18).

will be able to advise you on standard rates for common procedures.

You also need to ensure that the dentist is scrupulous about sterile working conditions. Gloves and masks are a must, both for the dentist's protection and yours, and don't be afraid to ask how frequently his tools and instruments are sterilized. You need to be sure that your health is safeguarded at all times.

You should also ascertain whether or not an emergency service exists. While dental emergencies rarely happen, they are certainly a possibility, and a dentist who has an emergency service as a backup, or has at least considered what his plan of action would be in case of an emergency, is a good choice.

Finally, watch those leaving the consulting room for an idea of your dentist's skill: the expressions on their faces can be a good indicator of what to expect in the consultation!

RIGHT *The dentist's chair can be a source of great anxiety for some people. If you fear visits to your dentist, choose one who makes you feel relaxed and comfortable.*

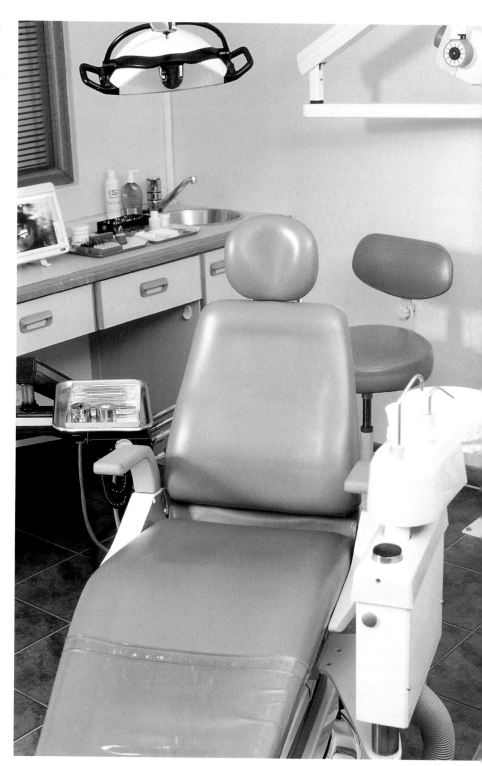

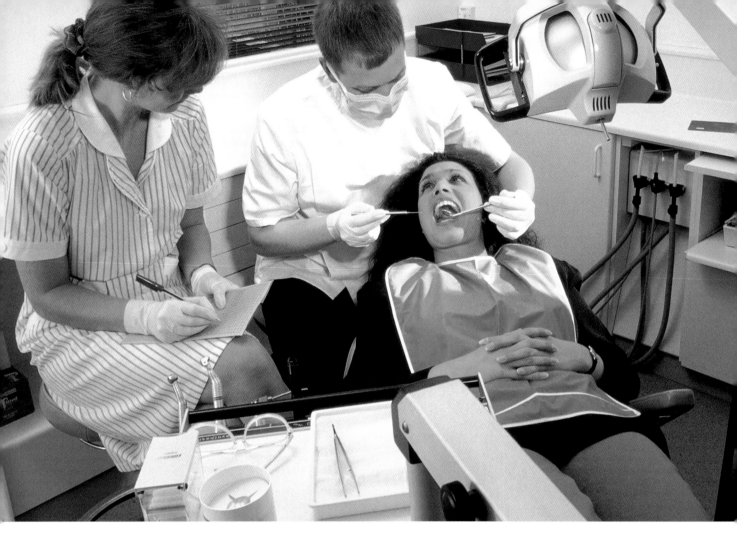

The dental checkup

As mentioned earlier, a standard dental checkup should take place every six months, and any additional procedures such as fillings or root canals, for example, require you to make additional appointments at a later stage. This is because many of these procedures take longer than the time allotted to a checkup. They may even require preparation time on the part of the dentist, or time between appointments for the dental laboratory to manufacture crowns and dentures, among other fittings. Consequently, if your dentist finds any problems during the checkup, be prepared to visit him again in the near future.

At the routine checkup, the procedure is fairly simple. Generally, when reporting to the dentist's receptionist, you are required to update any of your personal or health-insurance details, and then to wait to be called into the consulting room.

Once in the dentist's chair, you are hoisted up and backward into a reclining position, and a light is positioned above you to afford the dentist the best view of your entire mouth.

This is when you will be asked to relax – and open your mouth wide!

The dentist will take a careful look at different parts of your mouth. He usually starts with your teeth, looking for any visible signs of disease. Then, taking a probe, he examines the surfaces of your teeth, keeping an eye out for any discoloration, soft spots and cavities.

Next he looks at the gum area to see if there are any signs of infection or recession, or bad deposits of plaque or tartar. He also looks for any lesions that might indicate more serious diseases such as cancer, although these are rare and not worth worrying about as a rule. Overall, the dentist is assessing the quality of the gum tissue. Then, finally, he checks your tongue and palate to ensure they are healthy.

All of these procedures are completely painless; good news for those

who avoid the dentist for most of their lives out of fear!

The next step is X-rays that are really quite quick and easy, although they may cause a little discomfort. This is because the X-ray plates are placed inside your mouth, and you have to

OPPOSITE: *You can make a dentist's life much easier during a routine inspection if you cooperate and open your mouth wide when he asks you to do so.*
RIGHT: *Having your dental checkup is as easy as saying 'Aaah'.*

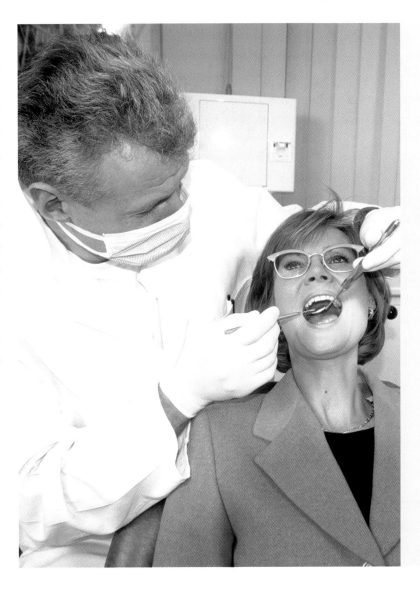

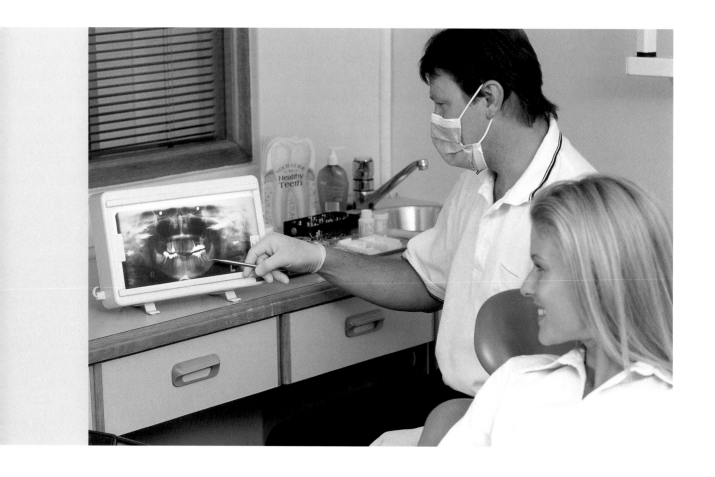

Your dentist will discuss any problems he finds on your X-ray, and determine the best course of treatment.

> X-rays are quick and easy, although they may cause some discomfort.

bite down on them to hold them in place while the X-ray is taken. From time to time they may feel uncomfortable, or may press on your gums or teeth. However, they take only a couple of seconds each, and are important for your dentist to be able to see cavities in your teeth, as well as the state of each tooth in its entirety, and the bone.

Once your dentist has checked the X-rays, his assessment of your oral

health is complete. Should you have no problems requiring treatment, he or an oral hygienist, simply cleans and polishes your teeth, applies fluoride and says goodbye until six months later. If you do have any disorders such as caries or gum disease, you will still go through the cleaning, polishing and fluoride routine. However, your dentist will also spend some time with you outlining the treatment plan and discussing your options.

DENTAL ANXIETY

Many people avoid their twice-yearly dental checkups out of fear, it's as simple as that. For many, this avoidance has gone beyond fear to what is commonly known as dental anxiety, where sufferers commonly spend a sleepless night before their appointment, as the mere thought of a dental drill can leave them shaking.

The consequence of missing your routine checkups out of fear and anxiety are clear by now: doing so only leads to greater problems in the long run as you will find yourself in the dentist's chair for long periods of time, and end up spending a lot of money on treatment for the neglect of your teeth – the very thing you've been trying to avoid in the first place.

Take a few minutes to take the questionnaire below. If you answer 'yes' to one or more of the questions, you need to work on your fears of

Many people avoid their twice-yearly dental checkups out of fear.

Take this little test to determine if you or someone you know suffers from dental anxiety:

- Do you often cancel your dental appointment at the last minute as a result of uneasiness and tension?
- Do you feel very nervous in the dentist's waiting area?
- Have you had unpleasant experiences during a previous consultation?
- Do you feel uneasy and anxious in the dentist's chair?
- Does the thought of an injection leave you feeling tense and slightly and nauseous, or even faint?
- Does the sight of a dentist's or oral hygienist's instruments make you feel nervous?
- Are you afraid or embarrassed that the dentist may say you have the worst oral health he has ever seen?
- Once the consultation starts, do you feel panicky and short of breath?
- Do you feel that your dentist is unsympathetic toward you?

appointment so that you can discuss your fears, ask questions about the consultation process and acquaint yourself with his consulting room. The idea is to make yourself comfortable both with your dentist and his surroundings, so that it's not all new when you arrive for the first time at your consultation.

Also ensure you understand what your treatment entails if you are having a specific procedure such as a root canal. You are far more likely to be fearful if you don't know what to expect, even if the gory details seem frightening to you at first. Allowing your imagination to wander without any facts will, most likely, leave you quaking, whereas the correct information is more likely to have the opposite effect.

Another option is to actively seek out dentists who see many children. Dentists popular with children tend to be much more patient and understanding with fearful adults.

Then, watch what you eat before your appointment. If you eat high-protein foods, such as cheese, one hour before the consultation, and avoid caffeine for at least six hours before, you'll be amazed at how much calmer you are. Sugary foods

Sweet treats before your dental visit will increase your agitation. For a calming effect, aim for protein-rich foods instead.

dentistry, and there are a number of ways you can do that.

Start by choosing a dentist you can really relate to, and who is understanding about your fears. He should make you feel comfortable and secure from the minute you walk into the consulting room. If possible, try to interview him (*see* p32) before your can increase your agitation, whereas protein-rich foods are calming.

The next strategy sounds obvious, but you need to breathe! When people are anxious they tend to either hold their breath or take short, shallow breaths instead of breathing deeply and rhythmically. Also, holding your breath decreases oxygen levels in your blood, thereby increasing feelings of panic, so it's vital to focus on breathing, and to do so in a regular, slow, deep fashion. Try to imagine your abdomen as a box that starts at your armpits and extends down to your hip bones, and then try and breathe air into the bottom of the box without raising your shoulders. This is a particularly good way of calming yourself down in any situation.

Finally, be creative about relaxation: either go on a course that offers relaxation techniques such as deep breathing or visualization, or pick up a book at the local bookstore or library on the wide range of relaxation methods available to the public. Alternatively, if you know that music relaxes you, take your favourite CD along with you to the consultation and ask your dentist to play it for you. You can even take along your portable CD player if he doesn't have one in the room.

If you've done all that and still find yourself tensing up in the dentist's chair, take a very deep breath and consciously relax every muscle in your body: tackle them one by one if you have to. When your body is relaxed, it is very difficult for you to remain anxious.

Most importantly, remember to be upfront with your dentist and relay your fears to him – he may well also have a few ideas on how to ease your anxiety.

Take a favourite CD along to the consultation and ask your dentist to play it to you.

Relaxation exercises and visualization techniques can help you overcome any anxiety you feel about visiting the dentist.

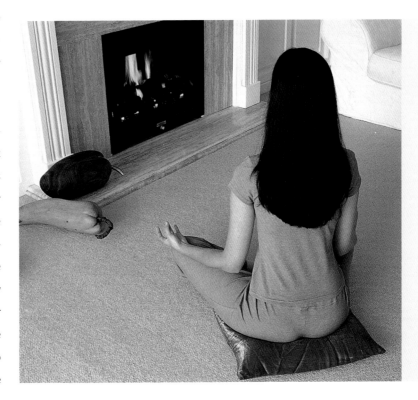

Common procedures

There are a number of procedures your dentist might use on your teeth depending on their condition. Obviously one should aim to be disease-free, but that's something of a pipe dream. The truth is that most of us will need one or other dental procedures at some stage, so here's a guide for easy reference.

Second to root-canal treatment, fillings are probably the most common procedure your dentist will perform on your teeth, usually to stop caries in its tracks. Most dentists will automatically use amalgam fillings unless you specifically request another kind, so it is worthwhile knowing what is available.

Fillings are the most common procedure your dentist will perform on your teeth to stop caries in its tracks.

There are, however, a number of other procedures such as crowning and tooth extractions that might be required, depending on the state of your teeth. It will be worth knowing a bit about these, both to allay any fears you might have, and to allow you to make an informed decision about the various options available to you. Understanding your options makes the whole process a lot easier to navigate: here are the basics.

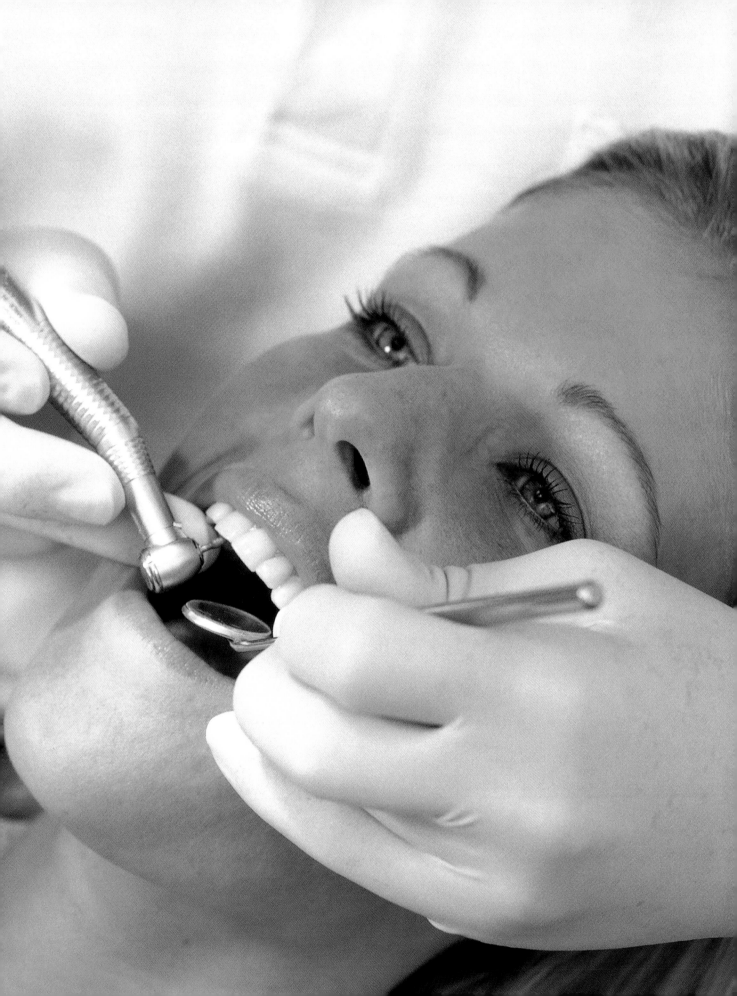

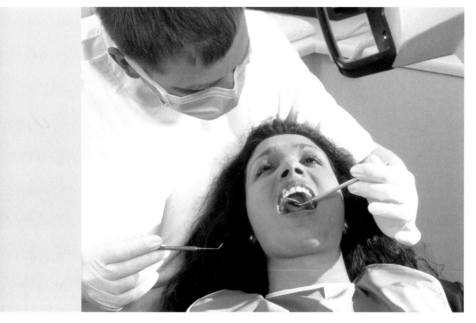

Your dentist first prepares your teeth and administers an anaesthetic injection before drilling and then inserting a filling into your tooth.

FILLINGS

Be aware that most fillings require a local anaesthetic injection in the area around the affected tooth, which leaves one side of your mouth feeling numb for a couple of hours. You can ask the dentist not to give you an injection, but then you have to put up with any accompanying pain.

Fissure sealants

There's one sort of filling your dentist can insert without you having developed any cavities: a fissure sealant. These are preventive fillings that can reduce the incidence of caries by up to 80 per cent.

Many people have deep grooves or fissures in their molars and premolars, and even though they are deep enough to cause problems, they are also very narrow and virtually impossible to clean. Some may be smaller than a single bristle on your toothbrush, and yet that's just enough of a gap in your teeth to allow food to accumulate and plaque to form.

Fissure sealants fill all these tiny spaces, and therefore prevent food from lodging in them. Obviously, this then reduces your risk of dental caries. The procedure is totally painless, and the sealants last for a good number of years.

Sealants can only be applied to the chewing surfaces of teeth, not the areas between teeth. They can be used on children as young as three or four years of age, on both the primary molars, and on permanent molars as soon as they erupt, initially at age six, then around age 10 through to the mid-teens.

The teeth are sealed as follows: first the fissure is thoroughly cleaned with the aid of drills and brushes, then the enamel is microscopically roughened by a swab dipped in acid. This allows the sealant to stick well to the tooth, just as you might roughen the surface of a piece of wood or metal if you were gluing something for a DIY project.

Next, the tooth is rinsed and dried, and the sealant is applied to the tooth and left to harden. It's a simple procedure, and an efficient way of preventing tooth decay. You simply need to ensure your dentist replaces the sealant when it becomes worn.

Composite resins

Composite resins or white fillings are mostly used in restoring broken or decayed front teeth. The dentist starts by removing the caries with a special tool called a burr. Once the tooth is free of any trace of decay, a protective layer is applied over the area to prevent the tooth becoming

sensitive, and then the enamel is roughened with a weak acid, as in the fissure-sealant procedure. This roughening allows bonding materials to adhere firmly to the tooth and ensures that the filling stays in its place.

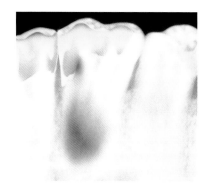

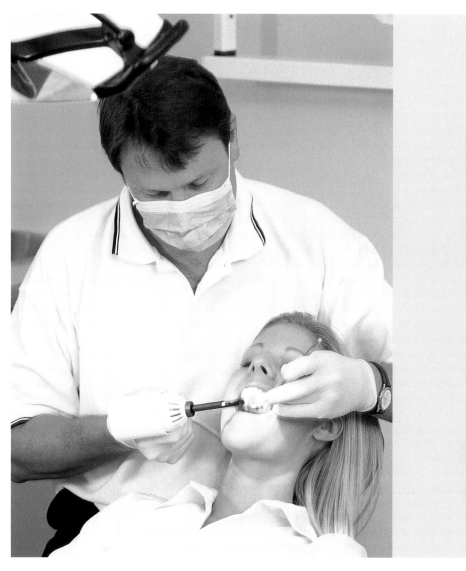

TOP RIGHT: *Many patients are opting to replace their outdated gold fillings with composite resin, which leaves them with a natural-looking smile.*
RIGHT: *The dentist removes all traces of caries before curing a composite resin onto the cavity.*

Next, after the tooth has been rinsed and dried, a bonding material is applied, and the colour-matched resin is placed onto the prepared area. While holding the resin in position, the dentist then hardens it using a special light. Once hard, the resin is smoothed off and well polished.

This technique is used mainly for smaller fillings. If, however, the cavity is quite large, a steel pin may be inserted into the tooth as extra support for the filling. Once the caries has been removed as above, the dentist creates a bevelled edge around the area to ensure a stronger bond. The bevelled edge is a slight indentation around the area on the tooth that allows the resin to fit more snugly. The dentine is again covered with a protective lining and the dentist then drills a pilot hole into the tooth itself. A small pin is screwed into the hole, and the resin is applied to the pin and the surface around it, and finished as described above.

Amalgam fillings

Amalgam fillings are the ones most of us are familiar with; they are a silver-black colour and have been around for years. They are also very controversial because they contain mercury,

one of the most toxic chemical elements known to man, but more about that later. Let's first look at how the amalgam fillings are inserted.

First your dentist removes any signs of caries with a drill, and then applies a protective lining to the dentine of the tooth. Often, a flexible band that simulates the natural shape and contour of your tooth is then positioned around it to help the amalgam take on the correct shape. The amalgam is then mixed, inserted into the prepared cavity, and thoroughly compressed. You feel some pushing down onto the tooth and gum, but otherwise the discomfort is minimal.

Any excess amalgam is then removed, as is the band, and the filling is smoothed. You need to bear in mind that an amalgam filling only attains its full strength after 24 hours, so it's vital that you do not chew on it immediately, to allow it to set properly. For this reason, it also cannot be polished at the consultation, so your dentist will polish it up the next time you visit.

Amalgam fillings may also require reinforcement by means of a pin. Once your dentist has cleaned and lined the tooth as above, a pin is inserted into the tooth using a special

An amalgam filling only attains its full strength after 24 hours of being mixed, so it's vital you do not chew on it immediately after your visit.

drill. The band is then put onto the tooth, the amalgam is inserted, and, once the band has been removed, the filling is contoured so that it is comfortable when you bite or chew.

The amalgam debate

Every couple of years or so, there's a resurgence of the outcry against amalgam fillings. All kinds of claims have been made about amalgam, citing it as the cause of a number of medical conditions. The list is long, and includes everything from memory loss and fibromyalgia to gum disease and even insomnia. So, what's it all about?

Let's start by looking at what amalgam is. It consists of different metals such as silver, copper and tin, to which mercury has been added: a mixture that has been used to make dental amalgam for more than a century. The mercury bonds the metals chemically into a hard, stable, restorative material that is highly durable. Amalgam expands and contracts with temperature change at the same rate as the surrounding natural tooth. It is also very strong, able to withstand the substantial forces exerted on it by normal chewing. All those involved in the debate are as vociferous as their opponents in either supporting or decrying amalgam. Both sides make good points, so it's difficult to get a clear picture of what the truth is.

So, here is what we do know: Mercury is highly toxic, one of the most poisonous substances known to man. Ingested in large quantities, over a long period of time, it can have a negative impact on your health. It's also something that's naturally present in our bodies; there's mercury in the air, our water, even our food. While the body's natural detox organs – the liver and kidneys – flush the mercury from our system into our urine, there's always a low level of it present in our bodies. Supporters of the anti-amalgam

Amalgam consists of different metals such as silver, copper and tin, to which mercury has been added.

Amalgam has been used to make fillings for more than a century. It is extremely hard-wearing and able to withstand substantial pressure.

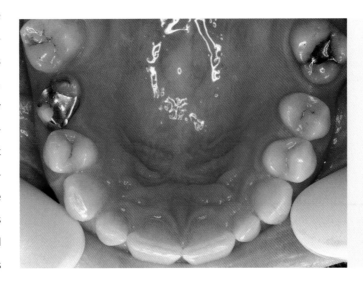

school of thought blame amalgam for a host of conditions, and suggest that simply removing your amalgam fillings and replacing them with composite resin, for example, can cure you of whatever affliction the amalgam is alleged to have caused. Unfortunately, all this is expensive, unnecessary and leads to prolonged dental treatment. In fairness, there have been cases where patients have shown a definite allergic reaction to their amalgam fillings, but this is extremely rare.

The dental fraternity has also investigated the safety of amalgam, and a number of scientific studies undertaken have been unable to show any link between amalgam and other illnesses. To back up these studies, the World Health Organization's 1994 Consensus Statement on Dental Amalgam concluded that amalgam fillings are safe and cost-effective, but conceded that there was an extremely low risk of allergic reaction or side effects in the odd patient.

It's difficult to decide who's right, but the bottom line is this: if you're worried about any possible side-effects of amalgam fillings in your teeth, ask your dentist to use a different material next time you have a fill-

ing. You can even have old amalgam fillings removed and replaced; just take into account the cost of the procedure and the time you are likely to spend in the dentist's chair.

Cast fillings

Amalgam or composite resin fillings are soft when inserted into the tooth, and only harden later. As a result, these are suited to small cavities.

If, however, you have a large cavity, with little tooth remaining, it may be necessary for your dentist to insert a precast filling. These are usually made out of gold or fired porcelain, and are hardened prior to being placed onto the tooth, as their name suggests. These not only fill the hole that the caries has left, but give the remaining tooth extra support.

ROOT-CANAL TREATMENT

This is the treatment most people seem to fear the most, because it involves removing the nerve and blood vessels that supply the tooth. Root-canal treatment is usually necessary because of deep caries, or a bad tooth fracture. This is because, in either case, the nerve pulp has been affected, and the result is really bad toothache and sensitivity to hot and cold foods. Root-canal treatment may also be necessary if you need to have a tooth crowned as it helps the dentist to gain support for the crown.

Once your dentist has examined you and determined that root-canal treatment is the way to go, you will have a good amount of local anaesthetic administered, to prevent you from feeling anything. First the dentist removes any caries, and then makes an opening into the pulp chamber below the dentine.

Next, using a very fine instrument, he locates the nerve and removes it, then cleans the entire nerve canal, right down to the tip of the root. Progressively thicker files are used until the nerve canal is thoroughly clean. Finally, the canal is rinsed and dried, and then filled and sealed with a plastic material.

It sounds quick and easy, but in fact, it does take quite some time, even if your dentist is able to complete the whole procedure in one appointment. Whether or not your dentist can do this in one session depends on the extent of your tooth decay. The key is first to clear up any infection in the tooth, and this may require a number of visits to your

ROOT-CANAL TREATMENT

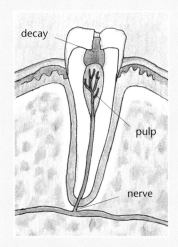

The spread of decay into the pulp chamber of a tooth.

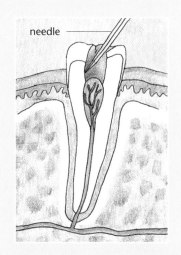

An opening is made into the nerve canal and rinsed.

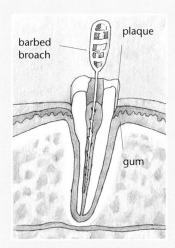

The nerve is removed using a barbed broach, and the pulp-cavity content is removed.

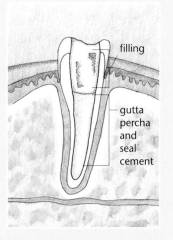

The nerve canal is filed down to shape and then filled and sealed with a plastic material.

49

Antibiotics may also be prescribed if your infection is very bad.

Also be aware that a tooth may have up to four nerve canals, and the same procedure may have to be followed with each of the canals, which takes more time.

Finally, do not be surprised if your tooth changes colour; a nerveless tooth goes a blue-black colour. This is most often why a root-canal treatment is followed up with a crown placement to ensure your smile isn't marred by the discoloured teeth that result.

CROWNS

A crown is a replacement of the outside casing of your tooth that is permanently fixed to the tooth below. In other words, the decayed or damaged area of your tooth is removed and replaced by a synthetic material, such as porcelain, to create a new 'tooth' with permanent results.

Crowns are often used after a root-canal treatment, because the removal of a nerve causes a tooth to discolour. However, there are other reasons your dentist might crown one or more of your teeth: to restore a damaged or fractured tooth, to protect a weakened tooth so that it does not fracture

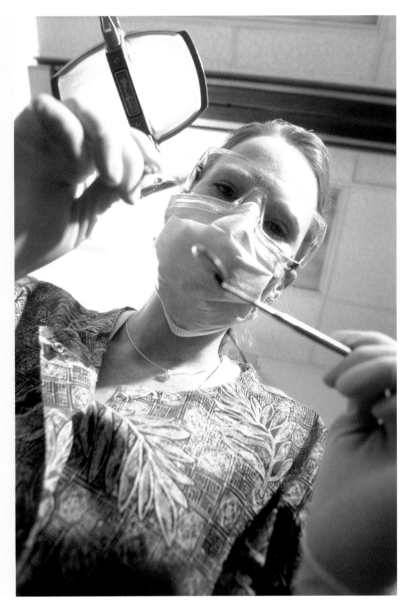

You will have to get used to this view, because root-canal work takes some time!

dentist, in which case he may insert temporary fillings in your teeth between each visit. These may feel rather strange at first, but are necessary to keep food and other debris out of the nerve pulp.

under stress or to reinforce a large filling where there is not enough tooth structure left below.

Crowns are also made out of various materials: gold or nonprecious alloy, porcelain or ceramics, acrylic or composite resins, or even a combination of porcelain on metal. Obviously the material chosen will be in line with what will work best for your particular problem.

When crowning a tooth, your dentist starts by filing away between 1mm (0,04in) and 2mm (0.08in) on every surface of your tooth, and then the entire surface is smoothed. Next, an impression is taken of the prepared tooth by syringing an impression material into the space around the tooth and holding an impression tray in position until the material has set. This gives the laboratory a perfect negative copy of your tooth, which allows them to make up the permanent crown. The dentist also ensures he sends the laboratory details of

Crowns can transform damaged and unsightly teeth and give you a beautiful smile.

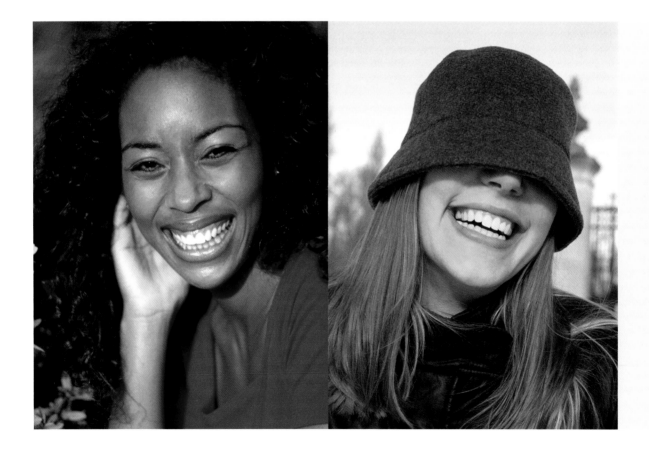

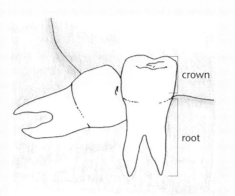

crown

root

Impacted wisdom teeth never erupt properly, which is why they often cause discomfort and have to be extracted.

extraction forceps over the crown of the tooth. He manually loosens the tooth, and then removes it. This is the most basic method of tooth extraction. Alternatively, he places an elevator between the tooth and the tooth socket, and carefully levers the tooth out.

However, sometimes it is impossible to remove a tooth using these methods, and then surgical intervention is required. Under general anaesthetic, the gum is cut over the relevant area, and the bone exposed. A section of bone is then removed to expose the root of the tooth, which is removed. Finally, the gum is stitched back together again.

Wisdom teeth

Wisdom teeth are the third set of molars that erupt in the adult mouth, and normally make their appearance between ages 18 and 25. However, in some people, they simply fail to appear completely.

If they are in a normal position, and functioning normally, then there is no reason to remove them. However, there is often not enough space in the gums to accommodate them, or they become impacted below the gum, and press on the adjacent teeth. Usually this means they cause all kinds of problems, including abscesses, periodontal problems and caries on both the wisdom teeth themselves, as well as on the adjoining teeth. This is why they are so frequently removed; as a result of the lack of space, they are prevented from erupting correctly.

Generally, wisdom teeth are removed between the ages of 16 and 25. This is because by this stage they have not had time to do any real damage. In addition, the roots of the wisdom teeth are still quite short. Once the teeth are fully developed, their roots are very long, and because they tend to grow sideways they can actually endanger your jaw's nerve system, as well as all the surrounding tooth structures if not removed in time.

Wisdom teeth are often removed in the dentist's chair under local anaesthetic. This is assuming that the teeth are easy to extract. In more complicated cases, the services of a maxillo-facial or dental surgeon may be required. As described, the teeth are removed under general anaesthetic, requiring a day's stay at a hospital or day clinic.

There may be a lot of swelling in the area afterward; because of this it is vital to follow your dentist or surgeon's instructions with regard to prescription medication and other vital precautions.

Remember to rinse the area as little as possible, especially on day one, and continue with your normal brushing and flossing routine without damaging the area that has been operated on. Essentially, avoid disturbing the clot on the gum. So, on the day you have the extraction, brush your teeth without rinsing, and start rinsing gently the following day, using a little salt water if you want to. Remember, that while some bleeding is normal, if you experience ongoing, serious bleeding, contact your dentist or surgeon urgently.

If you experience ongoing, serious oral bleeding, contact your dentist or oral hygienist urgently.

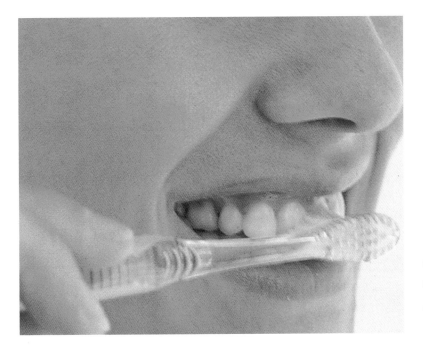

You can brush and floss as you normally would after you have had a tooth extracted, but avoid vigorous rinsing until the following day.

Children's teeth

Most parents, if asked about their children's oral health, would probably say that teething is of primary concern. From the age of about six months to three years, children get their primary dentition, or milk teeth, and it's rather a traumatic time for parents. This is because, while some children seem to get their teeth without too much bother, the majority of them seem to suffer from at least some pain and discomfort, if not a host of other symptoms.

However, there is more to children's oral health than teething and once their first teeth have erupted, they need to implement a daily brushing regimen, as well as twice-yearly visits to the dentist. In addition, children's teeth are far more at risk of decay than adult teeth, and may suffer trauma as a result of sporting or even play activities. Therefore, it's vital to understand the oral-health needs of your children as they develop. It's also important to teach children the importance of good oral hygiene while they are young, so that it is a natural habit by the time they are adults.

There is more to children's oral health than teething. It is vital that they get into a good oral-hygiene regimen early in life.

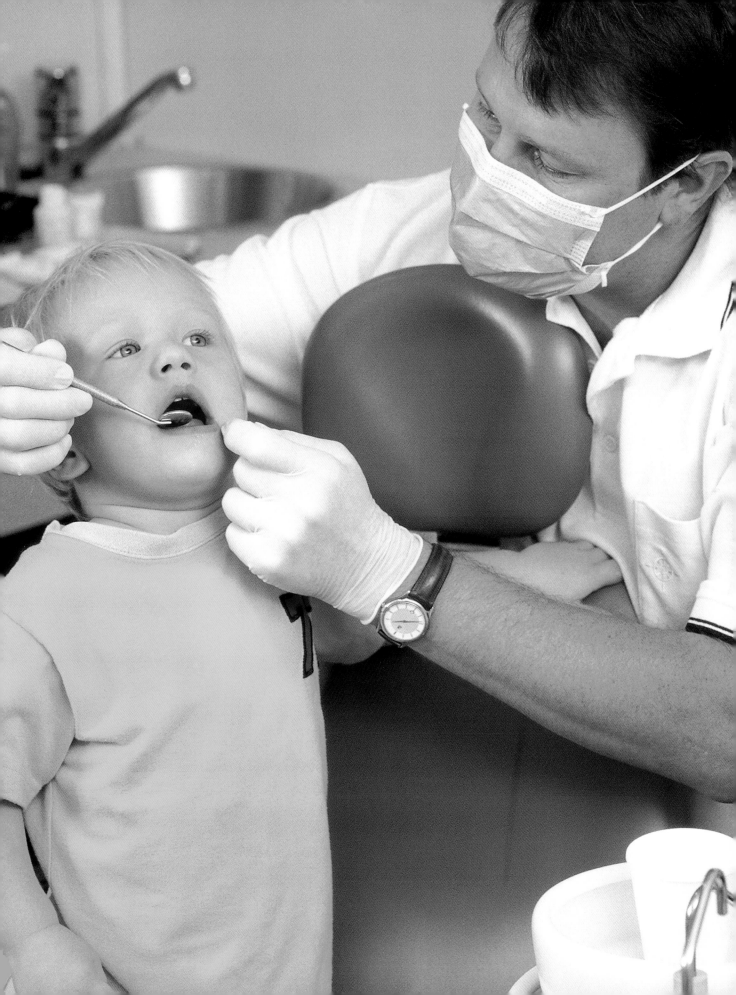

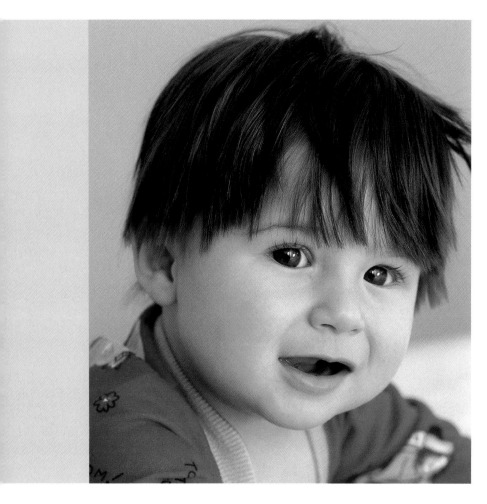

Teething is a very painful time for babies and toddlers and needs to be managed carefully.

TEETHING

Parents do need to understand an infant's teething process so that they can recognize the signs and symptoms of teething, and relieve their children's pain as far as possible from the start. While teething is difficult for parents to cope with because their children are so ratty and miserable, it's really far more unpleasant for their children. Apart from the pain they are experiencing, they often suffer a lot of other symptoms that can leave them feeling really uncomfortable and out of sorts.

The textbooks tell you that children's primary teeth appear in the following order: lower incisors, then upper incisors, followed by the first molars and then the canines. The second molars complete the teething process, usually by the time your child is three years old. Babies generally start teething at around six months, but it's not unheard of to have children who either start teething at four months and have all their teeth by the time they're a year old, or others who don't have a tooth in their mouth until they're two.

The key thing to remember is that babies don't read textbooks, and so, if a tooth pops up before you think it should, it's no cause for alarm. The others will appear in due course. Likewise, if your child is gummier than her peers, relax, her teeth will eventually make an appearance.

Babies show all kinds of symptoms when they are teething. Some symptoms are at the site of the tooth eruption, while others are so far away so as to seem completely unrelated. Firstly, around the gum area, where

Your child may be in pain when her teeth erupt, so it's important to remain calm and soothe her as much as possible. There are a number of things you can do to ease the physical discomfort she is experiencing.

the tooth is emerging, it may be red and swollen. Some children's gums even bleed a little. Occasionally, one or both of your child's cheeks may be quite flushed and warm, and she may be irritable or fretful.

Other symptoms may include frequent, loose stools, an angry red nappy rash, as well as a slight fever and runny nose. Some mothers even report that their children become exceedingly clumsy while teething. There's no explanation for this secondary set of symptoms, and doctors and other medical staff may be quick to dismiss them, but most mothers will tell you that they are very much part of the teething process, whether they make sense to medical practitioners or not.

A teething ring can do much to relieve a baby's discomfort.

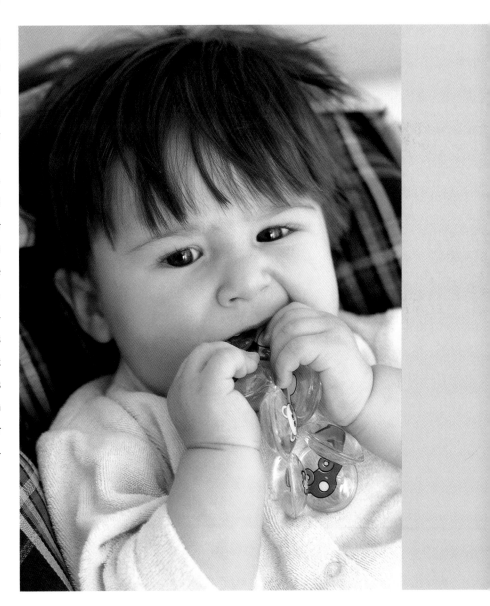

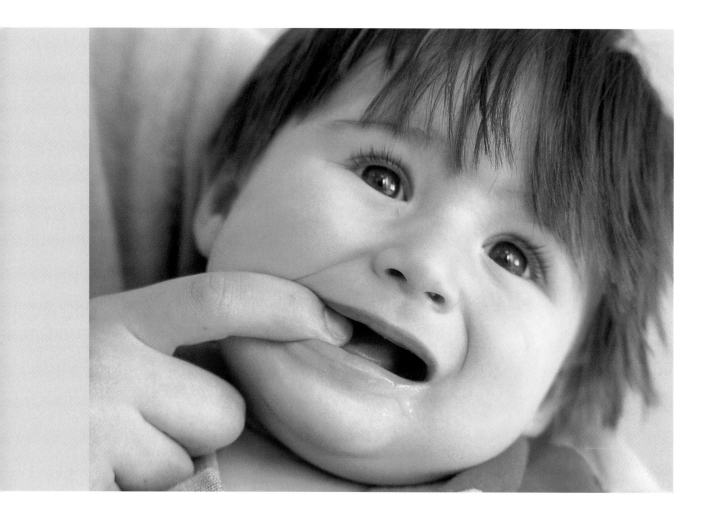

A little teething gel or powder applied directly to the gums will help to ease the pain.

Bear in mind that the urge to bite – and chew – is very strong; you can allow her to gnaw on safe things such as teething rings or large pieces of refrigerated apple or carrot. Toast crusts and hard biscuits are also good options, just ensure that whatever you give her to chew on is safe and age-appropriate.

There are also plenty of good teething gels and powders around, some available in pharmacies only, while others are freely available in supermarkets. You will find that your child responds better to a particular gel or powder, while a friend swears by a different brand. You may just have to try a variety until you find the one that works best for your child. All you do is place a small amount on your finger and massage it into your baby's gums.

It's also perfectly safe to give your child infant paracetamol to provide some form of pain relief. (Remember that aspirin should never be given to children who are younger than 12.)

Paracetamol, given at the correct dose for your child's age and weight, goes a long way toward helping her through this troublesome time, especially at night, when the pain in her mouth may keep her (and the rest of the family) awake. Your pharmacist or family doctor will be able to advise you on the appropriate dose. There are also some good homeopathic remedies available at health shops and pharmacies.

Finally, there's a good chance your child won't want to eat anything, but there's no need to be alarmed. It's not likely to last more than a day or two, and as soon as the tooth has erupted, her appetite will return to normal. Ensure she stays well hydrated by making sure that she has plenty of fluids to drink, and try to coax her with chilled, soft foods such as yoghurt or a home-made egg custard that has been refrigerated until cold.

CARE OF CHILDREN'S TEETH

Many parents fail to recognize that if their child has a tooth, it needs brushing, even if there's only one.

As soon as that first tooth becomes visible, you need to start brushing your child's teeth or tooth twice a day. These days it's much easier for parents, as there is a vast array of children's toothbrushes in every size, colour and shape, as well as brightly decorated power toothbrushes designed specifically for children's oral needs.

Likewise, there are many children's toothpastes on the market, which are usually fruit-flavoured rather than the traditional minty flavour of adult toothpaste. So there really is no obstacle to good oral health from the very start. You simply need to choose an age-appropriate brush for your child and start brushing.

Babies and small children do tend to swallow a lot of toothpaste, which starts to raise concerns about overdosing on fluoride. For this reason, ensure you only use a blob of toothpaste the size of a match-head for babies and toddlers, and no more than a pea-sized blob for older children.

The ideal oral-health routine is twice-daily brushing, but that's not always possible, as children have

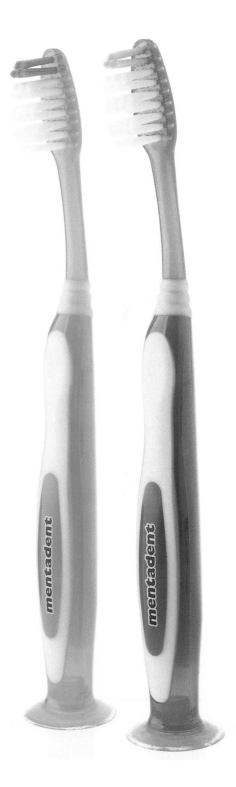

Children's toothbrushes are colourful and fun. Select age-appropriate ones for your children or let them make their own choices.

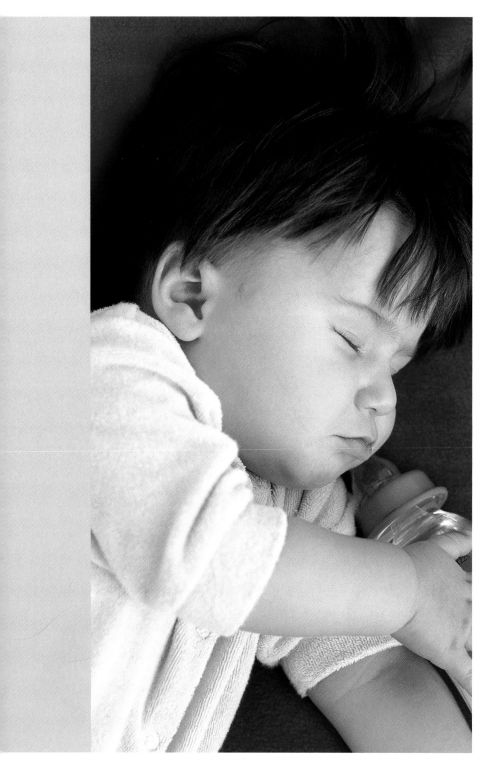

Avoid letting your child sleep with a bottle, or serve only water or unsweetened milk if he can't fall asleep without it.

minds of their own and may be resistant to having their teeth brushed. If you can only muster up the courage to brush his teeth once a day therefore, make sure it's last thing at night, just before he goes to sleep. This cuts down on plaque activity at night: you really don't want him to sleep with food and bacteria all over his teeth, as this essentially gives the plaque about 12 hours of uninterrupted time to do its damage.

Also, if your child goes to sleep with a bottle in his mouth, it really shouldn't contain anything except water or unsweetened milk. The sugars in fruit juice or other cold drinks will, most certainly, rot his teeth. Going to bed with a bottle is one of the biggest causes of tooth decay in babies and very young children, so if you can, avoid giving a bottle at bedtime altogether.

As your child gets older and becomes more interested in doing things for himself, let him brush his

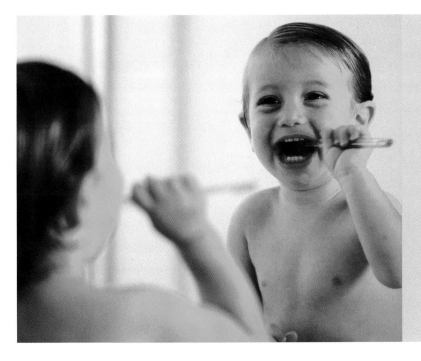

Teaching sound oral hygiene at a young age will ensure good habits for a lifetime of healthy teeth.

own teeth, but ensure you do a quick re-brush when he's finished, as he will probably just chew on the toothbrush and jiggle it aimlessly around his mouth. Realistically, you need to supervise his tooth-brushing routine until he is around seven years old to ensure he does a good job.

The primary or milk teeth are more important than most people imagine, because they keep space in the mouth for the adult teeth that are to follow. This is particularly important when the adult molars erupt. The primary molars are wider than the adult premolars. So, if the primary molars aren't there, the back teeth will tend to move forward into the gap. Then, when the adult pre-molars need to come out, there will be no space for them to erupt into.

In addition, children with a so-called perfect smile – where there are no gaps between the teeth – will probably battle a little when their adult teeth erupt, because there won't be adequate space for them. Also, parents shouldn't be concerned if their children's primary teeth are a little skew, as this is not an indication that their adult teeth will be crooked.

To prevent tooth decay and keep your children's teeth as healthy as possible, the same principles mentioned in Chapter 2 apply. Keep sugars and starches away from your child's teeth as much as possible. Remember these convert into acid that eats away at the tooth enamel.

Instead, babies and toddlers should drink cooled, boiled water between meals and well-diluted fruit juice or squashes at mealtimes only. Also avoid giving your child baby foods with added sugar, and ask your pharmacist for sugar-free medicines. If you can, wean your baby onto a feeding mug at six months as drinking from a

Avoid baby foods with added sugar and buy sugar-free medicines.

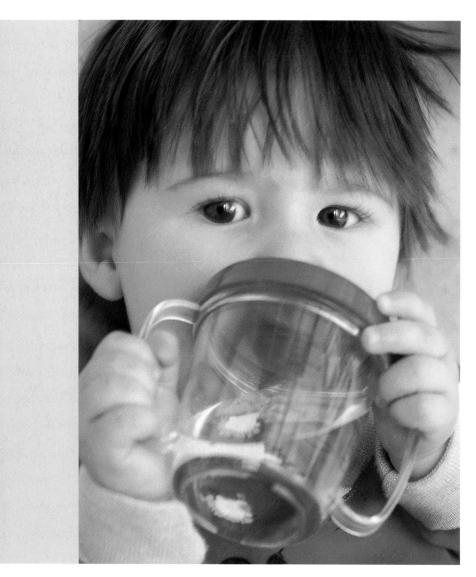

bottle increases the risk of tooth decay. Finally, if possible, brush your child's teeth immediately after meals particularly if they have been high in carbohydrates.

For older children, the guidelines set out in Chapter 2 also apply. Remember that your child's teeth are most at risk of dental caries, so if she subsists on a diet of cola and candy, she is likely to end up with a mouth full of rotten teeth. Countless children end up having their teeth extracted because their parents have not kept sugars and starches in their diets under control. Not only does an excess of sugary foods put your child at risk for obesity and diabetes, but it can severely damage her oral health too.

A feeding cup is better than a bottle as there is less contact between the juice and teeth.

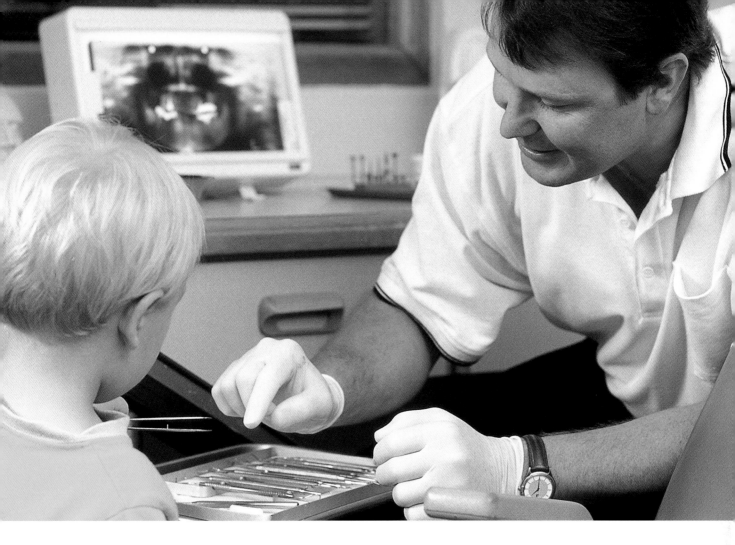

First visit to the dentist

It's very difficult to decide when your child is ready for his first dental checkup, especially when you consider the hang-ups many adults seem to have about visiting the dentist. Some dentists recommend a first visit when a child's first teeth erupt, but most will agree that it's impractical to take a six- or nine-month-old child to the dentist. It also seems a bit pointless to put your child through the bewilderment of a very foreign environment when, firstly, you are unable to explain adequately what is going on, and secondly, he only has one tooth in his mouth!

If possible, however, when your toddler is old enough to understand

Do not transfer your fear to your children. Create a positive first encounter by taking your child to a paediatric dentist who specializes in little patients, or find a patient and understanding dentist who won't mind paying a little extra attention.

Aim to make the dental consulting room seem more familiar, as well as a fun place to be.

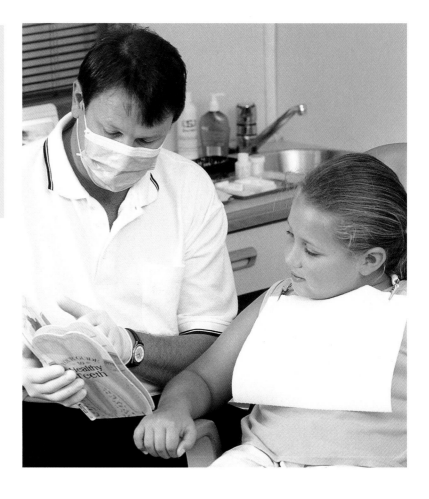

Choose a dentist who is sympathetic and has the time to explain procedures to your child in a friendly and non-threatening manner.

what it's all about, take her with you when you have your checkup. This introduces her to the environment and she's likely to be fascinated by all the lights and gadgets. Just let her sit on your lap, or even play on the floor next to the dental chair while you have your consultation. Then, if she's keen to do so, let her have a ride in the dentist's chair. The aim is to make the dental consulting room seem more familiar, as well as a fun place to be.

When she has all her teeth, at about two-and-a-half or three years of age, you could start thinking about arranging a first checkup for her, but ensure you explain what it's all about, and try not to scare her. Talk about why we have to go to the dentist, using children's books on the subject from the library if necessary.

Also phone the dentist in advance and discuss the appointment with him. Remind him to remove his

surgical mask when he greets her; a masked man can be quite frightening for a toddler. Also check that he has the same approach to introducing her to dental checkups as you do. It's very important that you understand each other, and that he has some understanding of your child's personality, as well as any anxieties or fears she might have.

Her first visit will, in all likelihood, last no more than about five minutes.

The dentist will probably give her a mirror and ask her to help him count her teeth, while he has a quick look-see, and he'll probably entertain her by moving the chair around. That will be that. It should get easier with each visit, as your daughter allows the dentist to do a more thorough check, provided you have a positive attitude toward the experience. If that doesn't work, a special treat as a reward for good behaviour works wonders!

INJURIES

If your child is involved in a contact sport such as rugby or soccer, where his teeth are likely to be knocked out or broken, you might want to consider having a mouth guard made for him. This involves a visit to the dentist: he takes an impression of your child's teeth and then makes up a rigid protective mouth guard that fits snugly over the teeth and gums to protect them. This really is a worth-while investment to safeguard his teeth for the future.

Dentists also happily make up bite guards for children who grind their teeth. This activity is usually reserved for when they are asleep, and makes the most alarming noise; it's likely to set your teeth on edge! Apart from the noise, tooth grinding can wear away at the enamel and weaken the teeth, so a bite guard is essential if you have a habitual tooth grinder in the family. Now, all you have to do is persuade them to go to bed wearing it!

Should one of your children's teeth be knocked out at some stage, and you are able to retrieve the tooth, go straight to the dentist with her, as the tooth can often be reinserted into the gum. Pick up the tooth gently, ensuring you handle it by the crown and not the root, then carefully place it in some milk or water. If neither is available, place the tooth in your child's mouth, next to the cheek, and get to your dentist within 30 minutes.

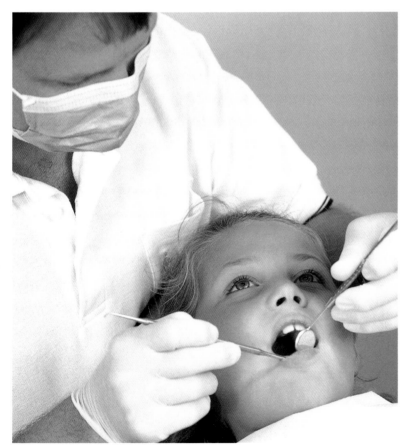

By the time your child is five or six, she should be comfortable with going to the dentist regularly.

A beautiful smile

There's no doubt that a beautiful smile can open doors for you; a mouth full of white, healthy-looking, well-spaced teeth can be your most attractive feature, and will almost certainly get you noticed wherever you go, whether it's in the world of business or in the social sphere.

Just as our basic body shapes differ, so everyone has a different set of teeth, and some people's teeth may not be as attractive as they would like. Perhaps your coffee or red-wine habit has stained your teeth, or cigarettes have left them with a nasty nicotine tinge. Maybe you have a large gap between your front teeth, or very skew incisors on the bottom set. Maybe you've lost a tooth or two through gum disease. Whatever the problem is, it has probably left you feeling self-conscious about smiling, and you would feel a great deal better if you could smile confidently.

Your coffee habit may be to blame for your stained teeth. If you are a smoker your teeth could have nasty nicotine tinges.

The good news is that there is a branch of dentistry devoted to helping you do just that – cosmetic dentistry – helping you make your smile as beautiful as it can be.

ORTHODONTICS

Orthodontics is the art of repositioning the teeth in the mouth, and is traditionally thought of as something only buck-toothed children go through. In fact, orthodontics helps a host of positional problems in the mouth, in both children and adults.

Take for example, someone with a large gap between his front teeth. There are several ways to close that gap, depending on what caused it, where it is, and the state of health of the surrounding teeth. You could restore the teeth through the use of a crown, or you could remove the affected teeth and replace them with a bridge or implants, which is clearly the least desirable option. Alternatively, you could reposition the teeth using orthodontics: the ideal treatment when your teeth are healthy and look attractive, because you don't lose some of the healthy parts of your teeth as you would during crowning. You simply move the teeth in the gums and put them in a more attractive position.

Orthodontics is mostly used for cosmetic reasons such as straightening teeth or closing gaps. You might have buck teeth, or you might have

Braces are not just for teenagers – they can be very effectively used to straighten adult teeth too.

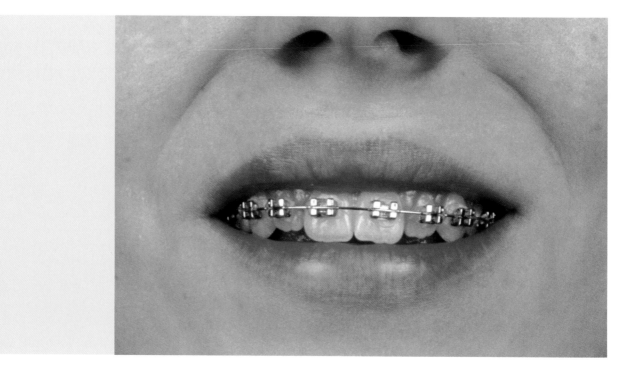

very skew teeth. Perhaps you have a gap that has bothered you all your life. If your teeth are healthy, but your smile needs improvement, orthodontics may be the way to go.

Many people may be a little wary of having orthodontic treatment, as we all remember a poor unfortunate soul at school who had to wear his 'headgear' for a number of months. The apparatus in question strongly resembled something from a mediaeval torture chamber, and was followed by more than a year of 'railroad-track' braces, and then a retainer. It seems like a long, torturous process, and the idea of battling with braces can be off-putting.

Orthodontic treatment does take a long time, there's no getting away from it. You're looking at six months to three years, depending, of course, on what your particular problem is, and you will require regular checkups and adjustments to ensure the desired result is achieved. However, modern braces are far less visible, and treatment may be as simple as a retainer plate for a couple of months.

These days, some problems may be corrected with lingual braces. These are mounted on the back surface of the teeth, and are virtually

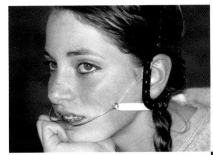

invisible. If those are not an option for your problem, you can also have clear plastic brackets fitted to your teeth instead of traditional metal ones, which also reduces their visibility to others. If you're worried about having to wear headgear, mostly these are worn at night while you're asleep and invisible to society in general! So there's really nothing to fear apart from a little initial discomfort.

Of course, there are possible complications, of which you should be aware. In some cases, the teeth move back to their original positions. This is the reason you are required to wear a retainer plate that ensures the teeth stay put after the actual treatment. In addition, loose bands on the teeth can create decalcified areas where decay can begin. However, this is not common, and modern bonding methods ensure the brackets are fixed to the teeth in such a way that the risk of decay is greatly reduced.

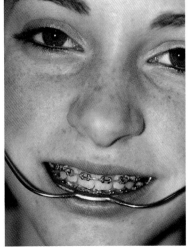

Many people put off having braces fitted because they are afraid of having to wear headgear, but this is usually only worn at night, and may not even be necessary.

TOOTH ALIGNMENT

An overbite

An underbite

Skew teeth

Correct bite

Treatment is usually performed by an orthodontist, someone who specializes in this field. Generally, your dentist refers you to an orthodontist, with whom you make an initial appointment, so that he can assess the state of your teeth and propose a treatment plan. It is a good idea, at this stage, to discuss cost implications, as orthodontic treatment can be very costly, and you need to know what you are letting yourself in for.

Your treatment plan may consist purely of braces and retainers, just retainers, or may even require that one or two teeth are removed to make space in your mouth. For example, you may have buck teeth in your mouth because there simply wasn't enough space for all your adult teeth in your gums when they erupted. To correct this, the orthodontist may have to extract the back molar on each side of the top set of teeth to make extra room in your mouth. This then allows him to move the remaining teeth into a more favourable position.

Also don't forget to ask the orthodontist how long the treatment is likely to take. It's a lot easier to put up with braces if you know when they're likely to come out. All in all, however, orthodontics is a painless procedure;

there is some initial discomfort from braces or even from a retainer, but this generally disappears after a few weeks. It's more a case of getting used to the foreign objects in your mouth than them causing discomfort.

WHITER TEETH

If you could see the damage your tea, coffee, red wine and cigarettes cause to the colour of your teeth, you'd probably embark on a whole new health regimen. Thankfully, they usually cause surface stains, which can be managed with diligent daily brushing and regular visits to the dentist or oral hygienist.

Sometimes, however, these stains actually go deeper than just the surface of the tooth. If you have tiny, microscopic cracks in your teeth's enamel, the stains can become trapped within the tooth's structure,

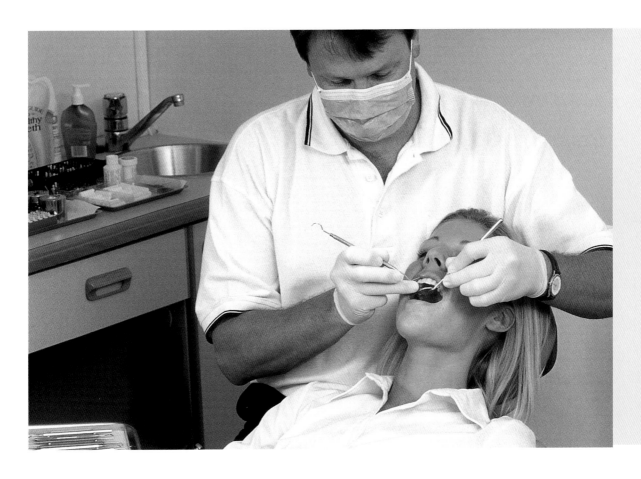

and professional cleaning alone will not remove them. Instead a more aggressive approach is needed.

Teeth may also become stained if you have overdosed on fluoride, as well as from use of a group of antibiotics called tetracyclines. These usually develop in people who were treated for some other ailment with tetracyclines while they were still very young – before the age of eight. They may even have developed these stains because their mother used a tetracycline antibiotic during her period of pregnancy.

Before you embark on a tooth-whitening exercise, it's essential to have your teeth professionally cleaned and polished. This helps your dentist to firstly, remove surface stains, and secondly, see what damage has been done. Assessing the extent of staining is important in choosing a correct treatment option.

Most people associate removing stains on their teeth with bleaching.

Tooth whitening can take some time, so get used to the fact that you may be spending quite a bit of time in the dentist's chair.

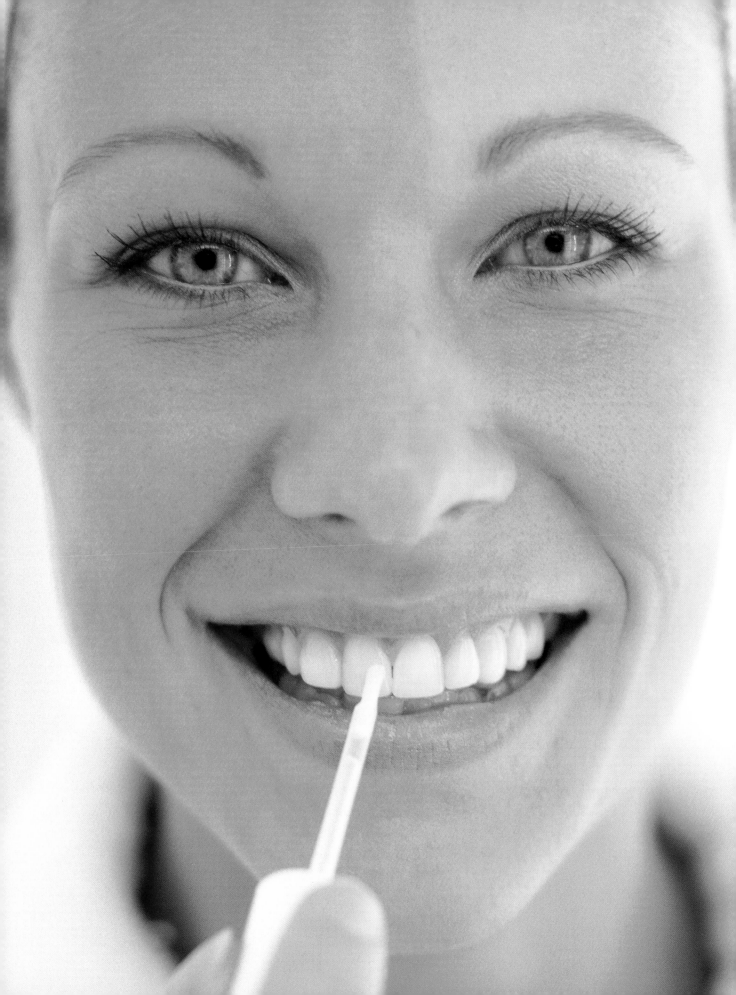

Bleaching works well in about 75 per cent of cases, and tends to work better on yellowed teeth.

You will have to play a part in the tooth-whitening process, and may be asked to apply an additional treatment to your teeth at home.

However, there are two other options if you don't want to go the bleaching route: bonding and laminating.

Both these treatments involve covering the stains by applying a thin coat of plastic or porcelain to the surface of the tooth.

Bonding, the application of a plastic material to the tooth, is a more conservative treatment than bleaching, and is especially useful if you have tetracycline stains, white or brown spots, or teeth that have changed colour because of amalgam fillings. Laminating goes one step further: a thin veneer of porcelain, composite resin or plastic is fixed to the tooth, and is very useful in teeth that have gone slightly grey, as these do not always respond well to bleaching. The advantage of both these treatments is that the stain is covered immediately. It is not removed, however, and the life expectancy of bonding and laminating is not as long as bleaching.

Obviously crowning is also a tooth-whitening exercise, as so much of the original tooth is pared away to make place for the crown. This, however is not a preferred treatment as too much of the original tooth is lost. Thus the most common way to whiten teeth for cosmetic reasons is through bleaching.

This works well in about 75 per cent of cases, and tends to work better on yellowed teeth. It is also interesting to note that cosmetic dentists tend to concentrate their efforts on the upper teeth, rather than the bottom set. This is because the lower set of teeth is more hidden, and is overshadowed both by the upper teeth, and by the lower lip in most cases. This doesn't mean you can't have both sets bleached, in which case it's advisable to do the lower teeth after the bleaching process is complete for the upper set, so that you can match the colour accurately.

To bleach your teeth, your dentist first separates the teeth being bleached with a thin rubber 'dam', much as one masks the windows, door handles and other accessories on a car when re-spraying it. Then he coats the outside surface of the tooth with an oxidizing agent, and exposes it to heat and light for about half an hour. It may happen that some of the bleaching agent leaks onto your gums in odd places, in which case you might feel a slight burning sensation. If that happens, point it out immediately, but don't be alarmed; your gums may turn white for a short while, but will heal well within a week.

The number of treatments you require varies according to the state of your teeth and the result you want, but you can expect to undergo about four to six treatments. Your dentist might also combine in-surgery bleaching treatments with home bleaching.

Home bleaching involves filling a plastic tray with the necessary solution, and wearing it for a few hours a day: a good option for teeth that are just slightly yellowed. It does take longer than the in-office version, but gives good results, is more convenient time-wise, as well as being more cost effective.

If you lose teeth, and don't have enough bone for implant surgery, dentures are an option.

Some countries, such as the USA, offer home bleaching kits over the counter, but it is advisable to consult with your dentist first to find out, firstly, whether you are a good candidate for bleaching, and secondly, which products are reputable and recommended.

DENTURES

Dentures are removable replacements for missing teeth and may replace all the upper and/or lower teeth, or just a few, in which case one speaks of a partial denture. It appears as though the demand for dentures has dwindled, especially given the introduction of new tooth-implant technology, but not everyone is a suitable candidate for implants. So, if you've lost all or most of your teeth, and don't have enough bone for conventional implant surgery, dentures are a good option.

If you've lost all your natural teeth, dentures help to keep your smile beautiful.

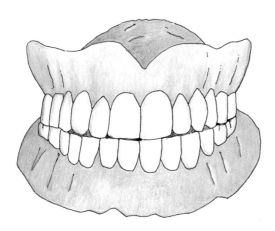

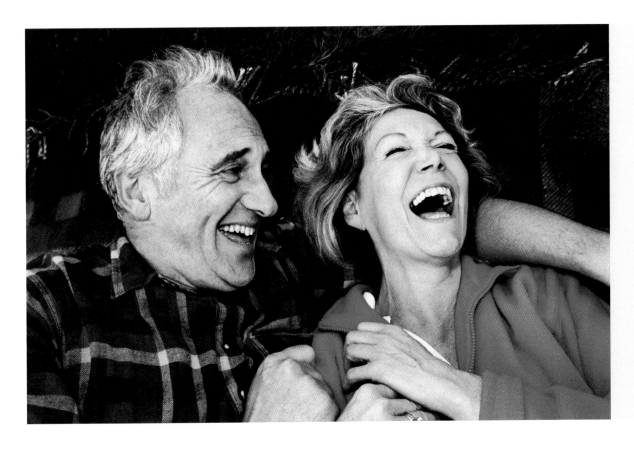

Simply carrying on with missing teeth is not a good idea. Teeth are vital for chewing ability, speech, and support of your facial muscles. Without teeth, your face also appears to collapse in on itself. So dentures serve a range of purposes.

Making up a denture takes about a month, which includes approximately five appointments. About eight weeks after you have lost your teeth, either naturally or by means of extraction, the wounds will have healed. Then your dentist starts the process. First, an impression and a wax bite are made to determine the vertical dimensions of your mouth, and to ensure the dentures follow your jaw position. Next you are given a 'try-in', a kind of demo model that helps you to determine whether the teeth are the proper colour, shape and fit. Finally, any adjustments are made and the final product is fitted.

It does take time to get used to dentures, as they feel awkward at first, and may affect your speech and eating habits for a while. In this regard,

Dentures help to support your facial structures – without which your face will sag and collapse in on itself.

When your dentures are not in use, they should be soaked in cleanser solution or water.

it's a good idea to start by eating soft, easily chewed foods for a couple of days until you get used to the sensation of eating with your new dentures.

Dentures need to be removed and brushed daily with a suitable denture toothbrush and denture cleanser. Dentures are fragile, so it's vital to refrain from using harsh, abrasive cleansers, as they may scratch the surface. You should also never sterilize your dentures in boiling water, and partial dentures must be removed before you brush your natural teeth. When dentures are not in use, they should be soaked in a cleanser solution or plain water.

It is also advisable to remove your dentures at night to allow the gum tissue to rest, and allow normal stimulation and cleansing by the tongue and saliva. This ensures good long-term health for your gums. It is also important that you visit the dentist every six months as usual. Remember that at the dental checkup, he examines your entire oral cavity for signs of disease or oral cancer, so for this reason it's vital you keep it up.

You should also be aware that as you age, you begin to experience bone loss and your dentures may become loose and uncomfortable. Do not attempt to adjust them yourself, as you can cause all kinds of damage to the denture and your mouth. Rather consult your dentist, who will either adjust them or remake the entire set.

There's also the option of mini-implants; these have been adapted from ordinary implants to help alleviate the discomfort of dentures. These mini-implants consist of a miniature titanium implant that acts like the root of a natural tooth, in combination with a retaining fixture, which is incorporated into the base of a denture. It's like a mini ball-and-socket joint. The head of the implant is shaped like a ball, and the retaining fixture contains a rubber O-ring that snaps over the ball when the denture is inserted and holds it in place.

Under local anaesthetic in the dentist's rooms, the mini-implants are screwed into the jawbone, leaving

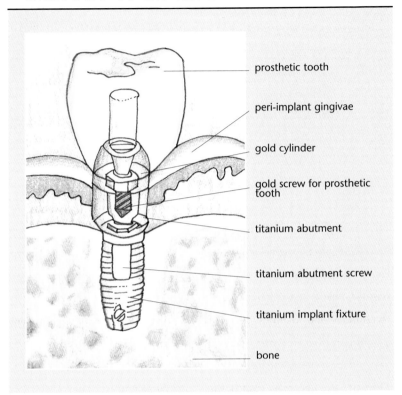

- prosthetic tooth
- peri-implant gingivae
- gold cylinder
- gold screw for prosthetic tooth
- titanium abutment
- titanium abutment screw
- titanium implant fixture
- bone

just the heads protruding. It's so quick that you can literally visit the dentist in the morning and be eating lunch with your new, stable dentures the same day.

IMPLANTS

When an entire tooth is lost, crown and root, shrinkage of the jawbone may occur, which consequently makes the face look older. Dental implants can stop this process. There are many ways to replace tooth crowns, as we have seen in preceding chapters, but only dental implants can replace the entire tooth. In addition, unlike dentures, dental implants look, feel and function like your very own teeth.

A dental implant is a metal or ceramic device that replaces the root of the tooth you have lost. Once it is secured in place, an artificial replacement tooth is permanently attached to it. Implants may be used to replace one or two missing teeth, or a whole

Mini-implants are designed to alleviate the discomfort of dentures, because these become looser as you age and begin to lose bone.

Your dentist will keep the impression that is made from your teeth for future reference and comparison.

mouthful of teeth, but it is important to remember that not everyone is a candidate for implants. Your dentist will have to determine if you are such a candidate after carefully evaluating your dental and medical-health history, as well as factors such as whether or not there is enough bone left in your jaw into which the implants may be inserted.

Implants are not simply inserted in the dentist's chair. Usually they involve a team of experts: a maxillo-facial or oral surgeon, a technician and a dentist, at the very least. Treatment also takes several months.

It starts with a thorough examination and X-rays of your head, jaw and teeth. Your dentist will also take impressions of your teeth and jaws to determine exactly where the implants need to go. Then it's into surgery, where an incision is made in the gum, the implants are put in place, and the gum is stitched back up. This may be performed under local or general anaesthetic; the latter is recommended if you are having a large number of implants inserted.

Within a few days of the procedure, the gums return to their normal state, although you may experience some swelling after the operation, and a soft-food diet will be recommended for four to six weeks thereafter.

The second stage of surgery is only performed three to six months later, usually in your dentist's office. Local anaesthetic deadens the affected area, and your dentist opens up the gum to expose the implant. Extension posts are attached, the gums are stitched into place around them, and a temporary tooth is placed in the gap you still have in your mouth. Then, about a month later, your new teeth are fitted. Some cases may require that they are fitted to a metal framework; others simply involve the artificial teeth being attached to natural teeth or being left to stand alone.

With proper care, you can expect your implants to last a lifetime, but good care is essential. Your dentist or oral hygienist will show you how to care for them properly, but again the key is daily plaque removal: brushing and flossing. You must also visit your dentist at least once a year for a maintenance appointment, which is an opportune time for your dentist to also check for signs of gum disease and oral cancer.

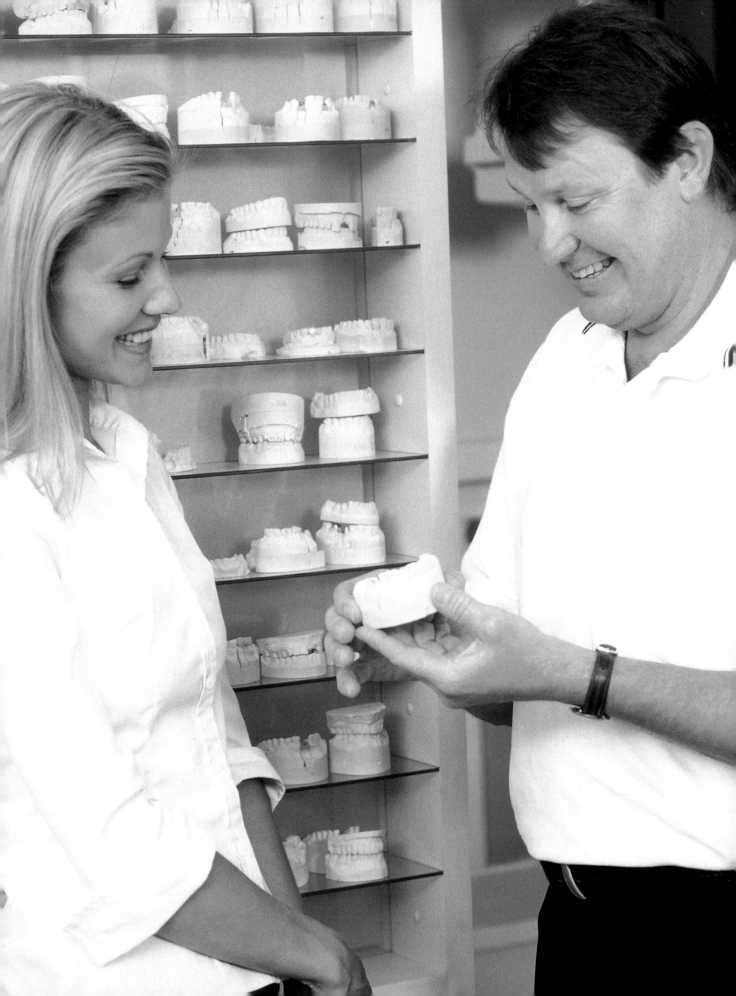

Further considerations

While for most of us, oral health is limited to daily brushing and flossing and visiting the dentist every six months, there are some people with special health considerations that have an influence on their oral and dental health.

There can be no doubt that lifestyle and genetics play a big part in determining whether or not you have strong, white and attractive teeth. However, should you contract a disease like diabetes, or should you fall pregnant, your oral health may be affected quite severely. It is important to remember that your oral health is a reflection of your state of health in general. HIV/AIDS, excessive stress, smoking, cancer, diabetes, even certain kinds of medicines may have an effect on your teeth.

Pregnancy can affect the state of your teeth quite substantially, so visit your dentist regularly.

For this reason, you need to ensure that you are living a healthy lifestyle and that your doctor and dentist are always fully informed about changes in your state of health. In particular, should you find yourself the victim of a serious condition, consult your dentist as soon as possible, to find out whether there are any considerations to take into account for the benefit of your oral health.

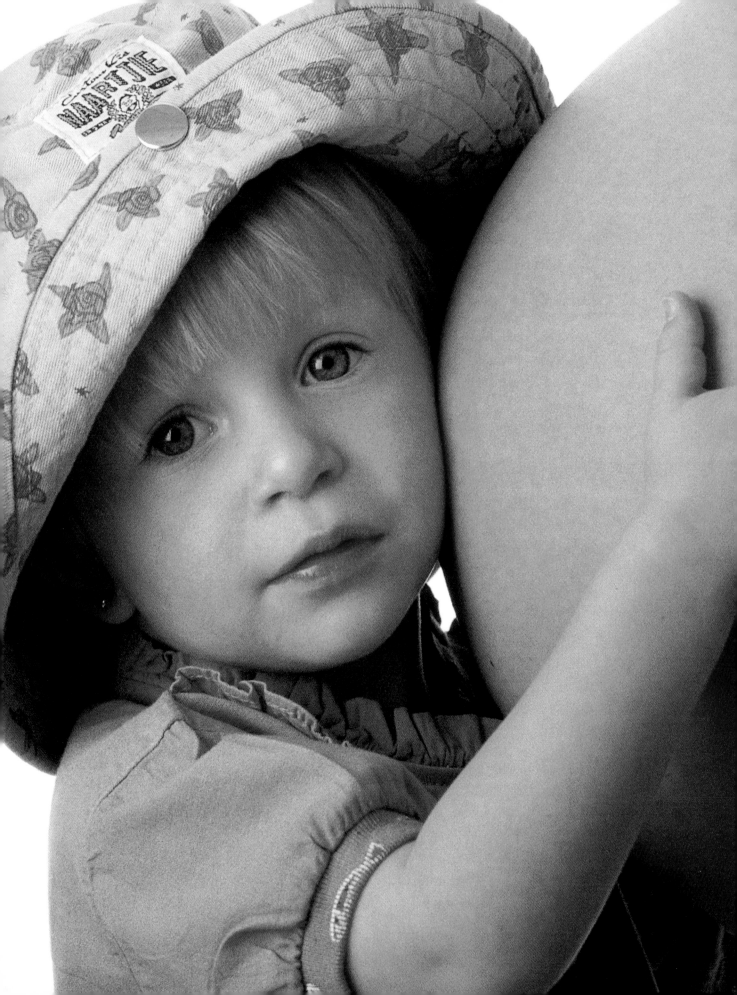

PREGNANCY

Pregnancy causes a wide variety of changes in every woman's body, and these often have a considerable effect on her mouth and teeth. There's an old wives' tale that one loses a tooth with each pregnancy, and while women will certainly notice a difference in their oral health during and after their pregnancy, there are a number of steps they can take to minimize the risk and ensure their teeth stay as healthy as possible.

The first factor influencing oral health is the change in a woman's hormonal profile, which not only gives rise to the mood changes associated with pregnant women, but also leads to inflamed gums. This inflammation causes the gums to swell, which makes cleaning teeth, and the important junction between the crowns and gums, more difficult. As a result, many women end up with pregnancy gingivitis (gum disease caused by pregnancy).

Pregnancy causes a variety of changes in a woman's body, and these have a considerable effect on her oral health.

Gingivitis tends to occur more often during the second trimester of pregnancy. This is because oestrogen levels rise, increasing blood flow to all the body's tissues. As a result, when cleaning their teeth, pregnant women often notice that gums start to bleed. This is not a sign that the gums have been injured. Rather, it is an indication that extra care must be taken to ensure that brushing and flossing are as efficient as possible.

Similarly, breastfeeding mothers should continue to monitor their oral hygiene, as hormonal fluctuations occur during lactation.

Diet during pregnancy is also an important consideration, because

Gingivitis is common in pregnancy, particularly in the second trimester.

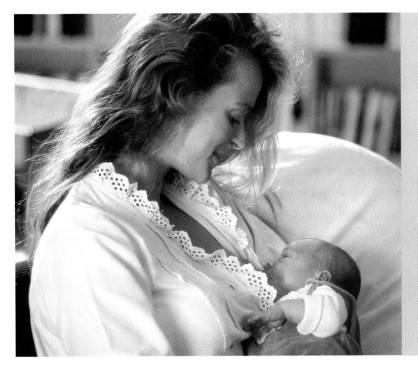

Hormonal fluctuations during breastfeeding may also have an effect on oral health, so continue to monitor your teeth and gums.

what women eat will affect the development of their baby's teeth. The primary teeth start to develop by the third month of pregnancy, and the permanent teeth that begin to erupt when a child is five or six start forming in the gums shortly before birth.

For this reason, it is essential that pregnant women take in enough Vitamin A, which helps to develop the tooth enamel, as well as Vitamin C, which is important in the formation of the inner tooth structure. Vitamin D also aids in the effective absorption of calcium and phosphorus.

Calcium is vital to ensure that a baby's teeth and bones develop properly. To make sure that the foetus is getting the calcium it needs, mothers-to-be should ensure that firstly, they are taking in sufficient calcium through their diet and secondly, that their body is able to absorb it into the bloodstream efficiently. Good sources of calcium are dairy products, as well as canned fish such as pilchards, sardines and salmon. The cooked bones included in the can should be mashed into the fish and eaten as is.

To aid the body in absorbing the calcium, expectant mothers should also expose their legs and arms to the sun (before 11:00 and after 15:00) for about 15 to 20 minutes daily. The

Mothers-to-be often develop bizarre cravings and eating habits, and may feel compelled to binge at odd hours of the day.

> *Oral cancer is the sixth most common cancer worldwide, and smoking is a major risk factor for the disease.*

SMOKING

The link between smoking and cancer is well known but usually lung cancer is what comes to mind here. However, tobacco users are also at greater risk of developing oral cancer than non-smokers. In addition, they are about four times more likely to develop gum disease.

Oral cancer is the sixth most common cancer worldwide, and smoking is a major risk factor for the disease. The prognosis for oral cancer is also not good. As it is often detected too late, only about a third of people with diagnosed mouth or throat cancer survive for longer than five years from diagnosis. Those who do make it have an increased risk of developing secondary cancers because there may still be cancerous cells circulating in their bodies. These patients also often undergo disfiguring surgery that is accompanied by mental trauma.

Oral cancer can also be malignant, which means it spreads rapidly from the mouth to other organs. Stopping smoking greatly reduces your risk of developing oral cancer: 10 years after you kick the habit, your risk of oral cancer will be similar to that of a nonsmoker.

of any medication you are taking. This allows him to choose the best treatment for you. People with diabetes have special needs when it comes to oral health, and you need to enable your dentist to make informed decisions regarding your treatment.

As a diabetic, you also need to ensure you take good care of your oral health. Keep your blood sugar within a healthy range, and take good care of your teeth and gums, ensuring you see your dentist every six months. Avoid smoking, and if you wear dentures, remove and clean them daily. The most important thing, however, is to ensure you eat the correct foods and take your medication as prescribed to keep your sugar at the right levels. This staves off a host of oral diseases and other complications.

Smoking also causes a wide range of other problems. These include brown stains and sticky tar deposits on teeth and dentures, as well as bad breath, among other negative consequences. Dentists also report finding small spots of white or red inflammation on smokers' palates. This is from the high temperatures generated by inhaled smoke. In addition, the smoking habit is a major risk factor in gum disease (*see* p26). It contributes to bone and tissue depletion in the mouth, and tooth loss is reported to be more prevalent in smokers than in nonsmokers. Dental implant failures are also more frequent among patients who smoke.

Many people who use snuff or chewing tobacco may think they are

The link between smoking and cancer is well known, but usually lung cancer is what comes to mind here.

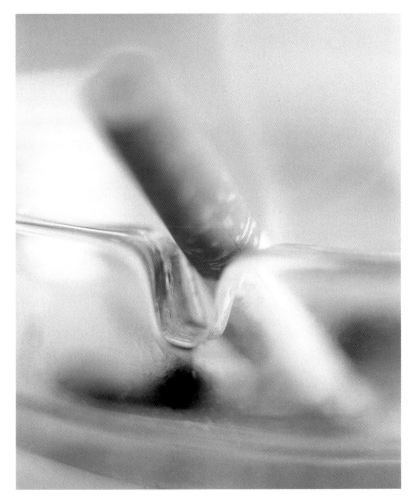

Smoking is one of the most harmful habits affecting dental health. It causes stained teeth, and can lead to an inflamed palate, gum disease and even oral cancer.

in the clear, but these forms of tobacco can be as harmful as the inhaled variety, causing an aggressive cancer in the cheeks, gums and throat. After just a few weeks of using snuff or chewing tobacco, patients begin to feel the intense negative effects such as stinging, bleeding and cracking lips and gums, and the development of sores and white patches where contact with tobacco is most prevalent. It is these sores in particular that are reported to become cancerous. Chewing tobacco and snuff also causes bad breath, tooth loss, a decreased sense of taste and smell, as well as stained teeth and excessive mouthwatering.

The bottom line is that any form of tobacco is extremely harmful to both your teeth and your general health, and it is absolutely vital you kick the habit.

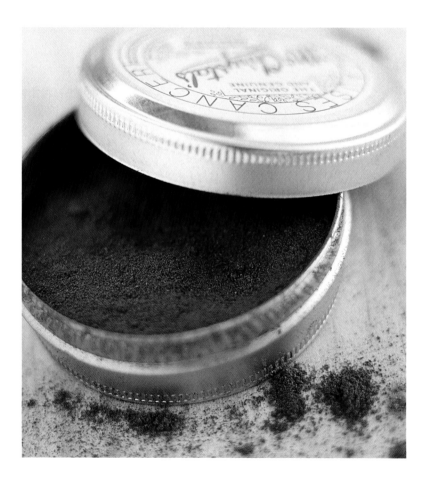

Snuff or chewing tobacco is just as harmful to your teeth and gums as smoking cigarettes or a pipe.

HIV/AIDS

People with HIV/AIDS are at a distinct disadvantage health-wise, because their immune systems don't function properly. This also has an effect on their oral health, as they are unable to fight off infections, especially if they are not taking Highly Active Anti-Retroviral Therapy (HAART) medication, also known as triple therapy.

Oral-health problems have two prongs in HIV/AIDS: they may be the first symptoms of the infection, but may also signify progression of the disease. There are some conditions more common in HIV-positive people: dry mouth, enlarged lymph nodes, oral thrush, hairy leukoplakia (a viral infection), Kaposi's sarcoma, swollen salivary glands, Herpes simplex virus lesions (fever blisters), human papilloma virus lesions (genital warts appearing in the mouth) and canker sores. Dry mouth is the most common side-effect of taking HAART. Unfortunately, it can increase your susceptibility to gingivitis and periodontal disease, as the saliva is less able to wash away the sugars, bacteria and acids in the mouth. To combat dry mouth and stimulate saliva production, use a mouthwash or chew sugarfree gum.

Oral-health problems may be the first symptoms of AIDS, but may also signify progression of the disease.

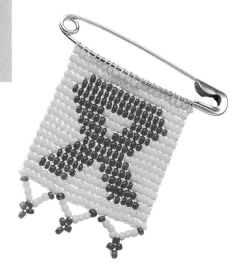

Oral manifestations of HIV/AIDS such as warts and thrush occur in up to 80 per cent of people living with AIDS. It is, therefore, vital that HIV-positive people are fanatical about brushing and flossing daily, as well as using fluoride mouthwashes or mouth rinses. While resistance to the disease is high, HIV/AIDS sufferers should continue to visit the dentist every six months. However, if the disease progresses and their resistance decreases, they should be seeing their dentist more often.

If you're HIV positive, inform your dentist of your status for your benefit and his. Your dentist needs to protect himself against infection; to know the stage at which the disease is, and the medication you are taking, so that he can tailor his treatment to your condition.

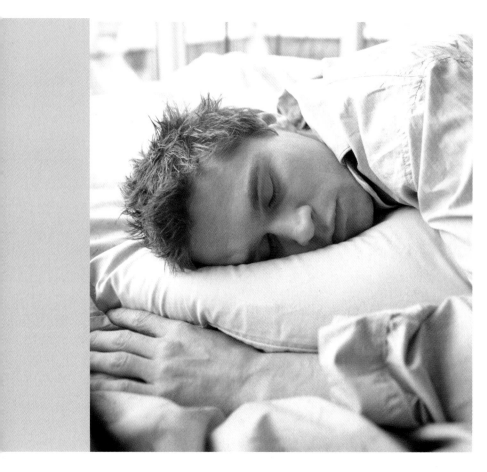

ABOVE *Grinding your teeth while you sleep may be a sign that you are not managing your stress levels effectively.* OPPOSITE *The stress of a high-powered job, as well as the other commitments in your life, can all have an effect on your state of health.*

STRESS

Most people would agree that stress is one of the major maladies of the 21st century – we all live very pressurized lives, and stress seems to go with the territory. While stress has its positive side, by motivating us and getting us going, it can also have very detrimental effects on our health, particularly if we are not managing it correctly, or we are overstressed.

Stress also plays a part in our oral health – many people, when under a great deal of stress, grind their teeth or clench their jaws, a condition known as bruxism. Mostly, this takes place during sleep and is not caused solely by stress; other causes include sleep disorders, an abnormal bite or teeth that are missing or crooked.

You'll know you've been grinding your teeth or clenching your jaw by the symptoms you get the next day. These include a dull headache or a sore jaw, and will probably occur when you are feeling the pressure at home or at work, and conversely ease off when things calm down.

The effects, however, need to be sorted out, as grinding and clenching your teeth can leave you with painful, loose or even fractured teeth. Your dentist will probably recommend a bite guard to protect your teeth during sleep, but you also need to find a way to relax and blow off some steam. Exercise, counselling, better time management and even physical therapy and muscle relaxants may help your condition. You need to treat the cause of your stress as well as the symptoms. Your doctor may be able to help you with suggestions on how to manage your stress better, but you could also consider going on a course that deals with stress management.

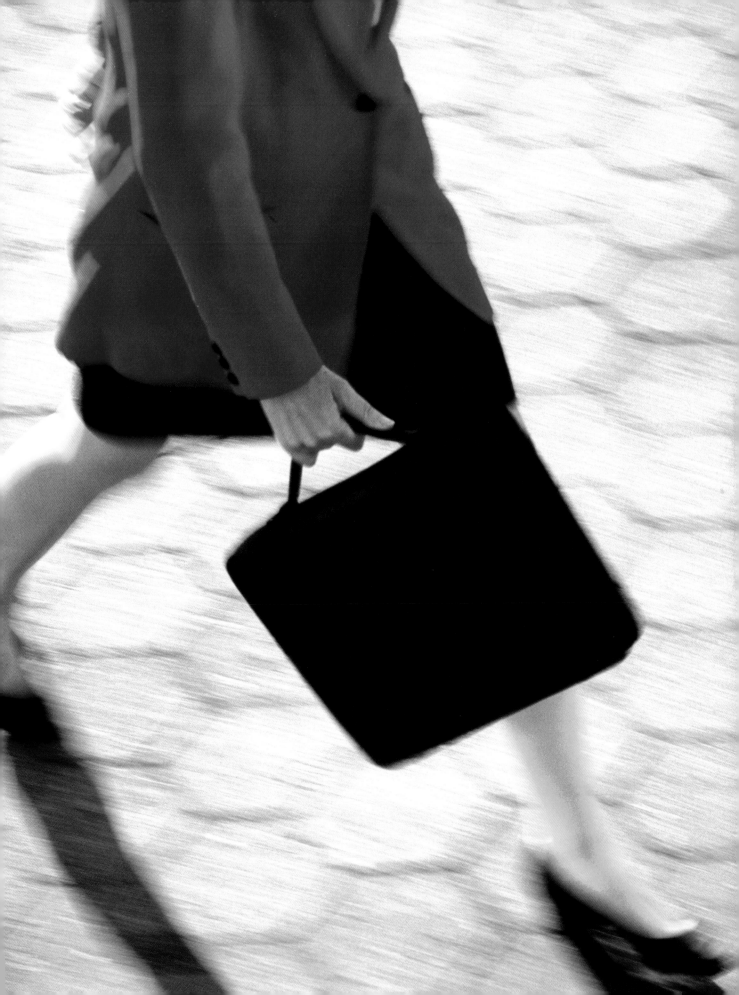

GLOSSARY

Abscess: A localized collection of pus in the gum.

Amalgam: A silver/mercury mixture used for fillings.

Bite guards: A device, similar to a mouth guard, custom-made to fit snugly on your teeth to prevent them being damaged by tooth grinding or jaw clenching while you sleep.

Bridge: A replacement of one or more missing teeth in such a way that the artificial teeth are fixed permanently to the natural teeth.

Cementum: A thin layer of bony material that covers the roots.

Composite resin filling: White, plastic-like material used to fill cavities.

Crown: The part of your tooth projecting from your gum. Also an artificial replacement or covering for the upper part of a tooth.

Decalcification: A loss of calcium from your teeth that weakens them and makes them susceptible to decay.

Dental anxiety: An exaggerated fear of visiting the dentist.

Dental caries: Cavities or tooth decay.

Dentine: The calcium part of a tooth below the enamel of its crown, neck and root containing the pulp chamber and root canals.

Denture: A removable plate or frame holding artificial teeth, which is a replacement for all the teeth, in either the upper or lower jaw.

Eye-teeth: The common name applicable to canines.

Fluoride: A chemical solution or gel that you put on your teeth to harden them and prevent tooth decay.

Fissure sealant: A sealant applied to deep grooves in the molars, which helps to prevent tooth decay.

Gingiva: The gums.

Gingival sulcus: The tiny space between the teeth and the gums.

Gingivitis: Primary gum disease that manifests as an inflammation caused by improper brushing. It is the first sign of periodontal disease.

Impacted teeth: A tooth that is not able to emerge from the gum and causes damage to the adjacent tooth structures as a result.

Implant: A permanent replacement for one of your missing teeth that is screwed into your jaw.

Laminating: Applying a thin veneer of porcelain, composite resin or plastic to the tooth.

Ligation: A process in orthodontics whereby an archwire is attached to the brackets on your teeth.

Lingual braces: Orthodontic braces fixed to the inner or lingual surfaces of your teeth.

Maxillo-facial and oral surgeon: A surgeon who specializes in performing surgical procedures on the jaw, face and oral cavity.

Mini-implants: A miniature titanium screw device fixed into your jaw, which helps to keep dentures from shifting around.

Mouth guard: A device used to protect your mouth from injury when you are participating in sports. The use of a mouth guard is especially important for orthodontic patients to prevent injuries.

Oral hygienist: Someone who works in conjunction with the dentist and who specializes in both cleaning and polishing teeth, and advises on good oral-hygiene practices.

Orthodontics: Treatment of malpositioned teeth and jaws.

Periodontal disease: Gum disease.

Plaque: A combination of saliva, normal oral bacteria and food particles in the mouth that sticks to the surfaces of the teeth, and in which bacteria proliferates.

Primary teeth: Milk teeth.

Retainer: A gadget that an orthodontist gives you to wear after he removes your braces. It attaches to your teeth and holds them in the correct position.

Root canal: The cavity in the root of a tooth.

Root-canal treatment: A procedure whereby infected pulp in a root canal is replaced with an inert material.

ASSOCIATIONS

AMERICA

■ **American Dental Association**

211 East Chicago Avenue, Chicago,

Illinois, 60611

■ Tel: +1 312 440 2525

■ Fax: +1 312 587 4735

■ E-mail: cherreth@ada.org

■ Website: www.ada.org

AUSTRALIA

■ **Australian Dental Association**

75 Lithgow Street, P.O. Box 520, St

Leonards, Lismore, NSW, 2065

■ Tel: +61 2 9906 4412

■ Fax: +61 2 9906 4676

■ E-mail: adainc@ada.org.au

■ Website: www.ada.org.au

BRITAIN

■ **British Dental Association**

64 Wimpole Street, London,

W1G 8YS, United Kingdom

■ Tel: +44 20 7935 0875

■ Fax: +44 20 7487 5232

■ E-mail:

enquiries@bda-dentistry.org.uk

■ Website: www.bda-dentistry.org.uk

CANADA

■ **Canadian Dental Association**

1815 Alta Vista Drive, Ottawa,

Ontario, Canada, K1G 3Y6

■ Tel: +1 613 523 1770

■ E-mail: reception@cda-adc.ca

■ Website: www.cda-adc.ca

NEW ZEALAND

■ **New Zealand Dental Association**

3 St Marks Road, Remuera,

P.O. Box 280 84, Auckland 5

■ Tel: +64 9 524 2778

■ Fax: +64 9 520 5256

■ Website: www.nzda.org.nz

SOUTH AFRICA

■ **South African Dental Association**

Private Bag 1, Houghton, 2041

■ Tel: 27 11 484 5288

■ Fax: 27 11 642 5718

■ E-mail: info@sada.co.za

■ Website: www.sadanet.co.za

PHOTOGRAPHIC CREDITS

All photography by Micky Hoyle, with the exception of those images supplied by the following photographers and/or agencies (copyright rests with these individuals and/or their agencies):

(**Key to locations:** t = top; tl = top left; tr = top right; b = bottom; bl = bottom left; br = bottom right.)

4–5	Photo Access	45	Chris Bjornberg/ Science Photo Library(SPL)	71 tl	Mark Clarke/Science Photo Library
22	Images of Africa				
28	Science Photo Library	47	(c)imagingbody.com	77	Photo Access
33	Photo Access	50	Photo Access	83	Lisa Trocchi/Images of Africa
34	Jodie Coston/Acclaim Images	51 bl	Photo Access	84	Photo Access
36	Photo Access	51 br	Photo Access	85	Photo Access
37	Photo Access	63	Photo Access	86	Photo Access
41 b	Nick Aldridge	70	Science Photo Library	92	Photo Access
44	Photo Access	71 tl	Mark Clarke/SPL	93	Photo Access

INDEX